INTRODUCTION TO HEALTH PLANNING

INTRODUCTION TO

Health Planning

DAVID F. BERGWALL
PHILIP N. REEVES
NINA B. WOODSIDE

INFORMATION RESOURCES PRESS/WASHINGTON, D.C./1974 I$\frac{R}{P}$

Available from
Information Resources Press
2100 M Street, N.W.
Washington, D.C. 20037

Library of Congress Catalog Card Number 73-87159

ISBN 0-87815-012-9

PREFACE

Increasing demand for health services, runaway costs and charges, limited resources, and cries of a health care crisis are making clearer than ever the value of careful coordination, cooperation, communication—in a word, planning.

Those of us who are students of health planning, as well as those of us who teach it, are acutely aware that currently there is little available in textbook format to guide and enlighten us in the fulfillment of our objectives as teachers and as students.

It is our belief that the diverse backgrounds, career experiences, and goals of our students, as well as of The George Washington University faculty, can be exploited to enrich the learning experience of all. Thus, for the past several semesters, we have recorded the formal didactic content of the lecture series for our graduate course in Health Project Planning. This material has been made available to students for outside reading and has formed the basis for seminars and discussions during the lecture sessions of the course. As our experience grew, these chapters were updated and revised and, ultimately, have evolved into this book.

The George Washington University Department of Health Care Administration offers graduate programs in Comprehensive Health Planning, Hospital Administration, Administration of Long-term Care Facilities, and Mental Health Administration. The Department uses an interdisciplinary approach for providing a balanced exposure to the areas of health administration and planning; urban studies; economic, political, and social analyses; and other relevant fields. Thus, all students study health project planning as part of the core curriculum, whether their ultimate goal is administration or planning.

This book is designed for students of both health care administration and comprehensive health planning. Also, it should provide useful information to those already working or teaching in the health care field who wish to consult a resource on the theory and process of health project planning. The literature in this field—which, of course, is still evolving—is scattered among many old and new journals and newsletters not necessarily specific to health planning. More new textbooks are needed.

We view this book not as an exhaustive resource, but as a starting point to understanding and skill in the health planning process, with some mention of possible sources for further exploration. We present what in our best judgment are the current concepts and issues in the field of health project planning. The structure of the book and how to use it are described in the Introduction.

Developing a textbook that will be of equal interest and use to many diverse types of students at all levels of career development has not been easy. In each chapter, we have attempted to acknowledge those whose works we have cited and those whose thoughts we have built upon. We are deeply grateful to all of these people, as well as to those not specifically mentioned, since our work is in great measure a compilation, analysis, and extension of the work of many. Footnotes, plus a list of references provided at the end of each chapter, will enable the reader to pursue subjects of particular interest in greater breadth and depth.

The authors represent various areas of individual expertise: comprehensive health planning, public health administration, information systems, community health services development, program evaluation, systems analysis and design, and marketing. We have gained experience in the teaching of health planning at The George Washington University through a team teaching approach unique in our Department. For this opportunity, we are indebted to Leon Gintzig, Ph.D., Chairman, Department of Health Care Administration, for his foresight in supporting the team approach and for recognizing, at an early date, that our lecture material might eventually become a text useful beyond our Department.

We are grateful to Ms. Betty Wright, Ms. Loli Malones, and Ms. Gloria Robinson for the extensive typing required in the preparation of our course materials and our manuscript. Also, we are indebted to Mrs. Viola K. Hargan for her assistance in editing the initial manuscript. We wish to give special recognition to the literally hundreds of students whose evaluations and constructive criticisms each semester have been invaluable in the development of this final product.

There have been a number of developments in the fields of health and comprehensive health planning since this book went to press. Some of the more notable events are the passage and development of regulations for Public Law 92-603, the tenuous continuation of the Hill-Burton and Regional Medical Programs, and the consideration of several national health insurance proposals. Also, there has been a major reorganization of the Department of Health, Education, and Welfare. This last event has resulted in the activities of the Health Services and Mental Health Administration—cited often in this text—being dispersed among several of the newly created agencies: specifically, the Health Services Administration; the Health Resources Administration; the Alcohol, Drug, and Mental Health Administration; and the Center for Disease Control.

WASHINGTON, D.C.
MARCH 1973

Philip N. Reeves
Nina B. Woodside
David F. Bergwall

TABLE OF CONTENTS

INTRODUCTION

Planning, a term which is widely used, is perhaps almost as widely misunderstood and misused. This chapter, therefore, will discuss what planning is, why it occurs, where it occurs, by whom it is done, how it is done, and, finally, how this book, with its relatively limited scope, fits into the overall context of planning.

WHAT IS PLANNING?

The word planning has many meanings. Often, in current society, it is a code word for public decision making; thus, we encounter phrases such as "the planned society." It is true that many public agencies are engaged in planning, but not all decision makers—public or private—actually plan. Planning, in fact, is making current decisions in the light of their future effects, and it is this meaning of planning that will be used throughout this book. The book itself, however, is addressed to the more operational definition that planning is the development and implementation of a course of action which is expected to lead to desired results given the occurrence of expected events; planning is making decisions now that will enable us to get to where we wish to be at some point in the future.

WHY DO WE PLAN?

If we accept the foregoing definition, planning would be unnecessary if, and *only* if, two assumptions were valid: first, that the world is static and unchanging; and, second, that our world is as it should be. Probably very few

1

nonplanners would be willing to accept these assumptions; nevertheless, they do not plan. Why? Perhaps they are convinced that the "unseen hand" described by Adam Smith does in fact guide the activities of mankind toward an eventual optimum.[1] It seems, however, that most people seriously believe that there is sufficient evidence to doubt the total validity of this concept. Consequently, if there is no unseen hand, there must be some mechanism to assure that our actions will be rational and efficient methods of attaining our desired ends.

One of the principal problems faced by the nonplanner is that most of his changes are implemented on a crisis basis. Because he is forced to react to whatever situation he faces at the moment, rather than to act on the basis of anticipation, he cannot influence the development of the situation to facilitate achievement of his goals. For example, consider a military commander who can either maneuver to force his opponent to enter battle under circumstances that are favorable to him or simply wait until he is forced to fight at a time and place convenient to the enemy. Planners need not adopt such a militant stance, but, in reality, they too are in a contest with external forces such as a competing organization or simply the constantly changing social, economic, political, or technological aspects of their environment. Thus, the decision maker has two choices. He can pursue, over the long run, a carefully devised course of action—calculated to take advantage of every opportunity—to influence the environment and to develop the resources required for effective action, or he can wait until it becomes necessary for him to take action and then respond—in circumstances which can be favorable to him only by chance—with whatever means he can contrive hastily from the resources that happen to be available. Clearly, the chances of success are far greater if he adopts the first alternative, planning.

WHERE DOES PLANNING TAKE PLACE?[2]

Planning, to some degree, occurs at all levels of human organization, starting with the individual and culminating at the national government. For our

[1] Both those who plan and those who make decisions without planning will agree that there are not enough resources to do everything that might be desirable. Therefore, the available resources must be allocated among activities. If the world were static and ideal, there would be no need to revise the existing allocations.

[2] The types of planning described in this section have been adapted from Jantsch, Eric. "From Forecasting and Planning to Policy Sciences." *Policy Sciences,* *1*(1):31–47, Spring 1970.

purposes, it is probably best to think in terms of a department within an institution or agency as being the lowest planning entity; the next level would be the institution or agency; then, a region or community that is part of a state, which, in turn, is part of the nation.

The predominant type of planning varies widely within each level. The first type is project planning—the major concern of this book. It deals with operational matters of a rather narrow scope, based upon problem-solving techniques and striving for efficiency. Project planning occurs at all of the levels described above, but it is predominant at the departmental level and comprises only a small portion of the national planning effort.

The next type, system planning, deals with longer range or strategic matters. It stresses the use of optimizing techniques that effect satisfactory trade-offs among components of a system, with the ultimate goal being effectiveness rather than simple efficiency. The system plan can integrate a multitude of project plans and make certain that the allocation of resources among them is for the benefit of the total community rather than for a limited segment served by some specific project. Although systems planning is conceivable at all levels, it is our belief that it would not be truly meaningful at the departmental level. Systems planning may have some use in larger institutions or agencies, but it becomes an important planning style primarily at the community level and above.

The third type is policy planning. This is a normative mode that stresses changing value systems toward the end of achieving objectives such as equity and equality. It establishes the overall context within which systems planning will take place. In particular, it leads to the development of criteria for measuring systems' effectiveness. Normative planning is most effective at national and state levels, where there are explicit mechanisms for developing and implementing the normative choices of our society—primarily through legislative action. It is not inconceivable, however, that normative judgments can be developed and implemented at the community level, although, in most cases, the mechanisms would be less formal.

WHO PLANS?

The preceding section has answered this question in part. It is worth noting, however, that planners at the different levels often serve in very different roles. For example, at the departmental level, they might be engaged primarily in productive or administrative functions and will perform planning only as an adjunct activity. Planning becomes more of a management function at the institutional or agency level and, in some cases, becomes the primary mission of one or more staff persons. At the regional or community level, we frequently find voluntary agencies whose staff members engage in planning—often with support, advice, or direction from a board or committee representing either the special-interest groups affected or the entire community. Within government, professional planning staff members can be found at local, state, and federal levels. Once again, these persons usually function with some type of board or committee whose activities quite often are supplemented and complemented by the direction and oversight provided by a legislative branch of government.

HOW IS PLANNING PERFORMED?

The specifics of how to plan a project will be described throughout the remainder of this book; however, a general approach to planning forms the model on which these detailed steps are based. Decision making can proceed through disjointed incrementalism, as described by Charles Lindblom,[3] or through a rational approach. Basically, disjointed incrementalism implies rather cautious movements from status quo toward the general direction that is thought to be desirable. Great leaps forward, based on a rational analysis of current and predicted situations, can be dangerous; that is, we are incapable of really knowing and understanding the situations and their ramifications. Consequently, there is a great danger that we will make serious mistakes because of our ignorance or misinformation. Incrementalism, however, despite its virtue of safety, is simply too slow in responding to the rapid and urgent changes taking place in today's world. Admittedly, the weaknesses of the rational model are all too real. Nevertheless, they are not as severe as the proponents of incrementalism would have us believe; that is, the rational model can be approximated even though we lack perfect information. Two of the devices for coping with our uncertainties and our lack of absolutely accurate data are simulation and decision theory.

Acceptance of the rational model as a basis for planning leads to the

---

3 Baybrooke, D. and Lindblom, C.E. *A Strategy of Decision*. New York, Free Press, 1963. Chapter 5.

identification of a series of steps required to carry out this concept; specifically:

1. To identify the desired state (set our objectives).
2. To determine the discrepancy between the desired state and those conditions that would be likely to occur if no action were taken (this involves forecasting).
3. To identify the resources that will probably be available to effect changes toward the desired state.
4. To develop feasible alternative methods for using those resources to effect the necessary changes.
5. To evaluate those alternatives and select the one that seems most likely to achieve the desired results at a reasonable cost.
6. To implement the chosen alternative.
7. To appraise the performance of this alternative and then make the necessary adjustments to bring it closer toward achieving the desired objectives.

Clearly, the above-mentioned steps are a highly simplified model of the planning process. Planning is not—and cannot be—a straightforward, sequential process. Instead, it must be regarded as a cybernetic system with many iterative loops; that is, at each step along the way, the planner must be prepared to review what has occurred in all the preceding steps and to reevaluate those activities in the light of current developments. For example, it is entirely possible that, in the process of identifying available resources (step three), we might discover that our initial objectives are either too high or too low. Should this occur, the planner must then go back and make the necessary adjustments to the product of step one and proceed again through step two to step three. This text will not, for purposes of exposition, restate the iterative process. It is the responsibility of the reader to bear this caveat constantly in mind.

PLANNING AND CHOICE[4]

The perceptive reader will have noted that there are three major points in the

[4] This section is based on Davdoff, Paul and Reiner, T.A. "A Choice Theory of Planning." *Journal of the American Institute of Planning*, 28(3):103–115, May 1962.

planning process described above at which choices are made; specifically: when we select the goals and criteria, when we choose the means of implementation, and when we redirect action on the basis of evaluation. These choices involve values that are not universal; consequently, disagreements will tend to arise. In the case of goals and criteria and evaluative actions, the disagreement tends to focus upon the dichotomy between consumers and providers. (Chapter 5 discusses this in greater detail.) The choices involved in implementation focus on means. In this book, we stress the economic evaluation of alternatives, but the other values that must be involved should not be overlooked; for example, whether a project should be a public or a private activity. The subject of public value development, however, is a study in itself and will not be discussed further in this book. We conclude by stating that economic choices must be tempered by values derived from the normative planning process, which provides the general policy framework within which projects must be developed.

SUMMARY

The emphasis in this book is on how to develop a plan when the planner also has the authority to implement it, providing he observes the normative values of the society in which he is functioning. Our approach describes a simplified, rational model and assumes minimum interactions with the environment and other components of the system in which it operates. We believe this approach to be very useful in developing an understanding of the planning process, in that it forms a base from which each person may develop his own skills in the more complex processes of systems planning and normative planning.

CHAPTER 1

HISTORY OF PLANNING

Writers for the public press and contributors to the professional literature have, for many years, called attention to the continuing health crisis in the nation. In 1849, Lemuel Shattuck, a Boston schoolteacher, writer, and publisher, who became interested in vital statistics and active in community health and welfare activities and who has become known as the founder of public health in the United States, wrote:

> The conditions of perfect health, either public or personal, are seldom or never attained, though attainable. Every year, thousands of lives are lost which might have been saved, tens of thousands of cases of sickness occur which might have been prevented. A vast amount of unnecessarily impaired health and physical debility exists among those not actually confined by a sickness, and means exist within our reach for the mitigation or removal of these evils.

Shattuck's report[1] on health conditions in Massachusetts, which was buried by the Massachusetts legislature at the time, included 50 recommendations of great impact.

A more recent report compared conditions of its day to those of Shattuck's time, and again some profound recommendations were made:

1. That medical service, both preventive and therapeutic, should be furnished largely by organized groups of physicians, dentists, nurses, pharmacists, and other associated personnel.
2. That all basic public health services be extended—whether provided by governmental or nongovernmental agencies—so they will be available to the entire population according to its needs.

---

[1] Shattuck, Lemuel. *Report of the Sanitary Commission of Massachusetts, 1849.* Boston, Dutton and Wentworth, 1850.

3. That the costs of medical care be placed on a group prepayment basis—by means of insurance, taxation, or both of these methods.

4. That the study, evaluation, and coordination of medical services be considered important functions of every state and local community; that agencies be formed to exercise these functions; and that the coordination of rural with urban services receive special attention.

5. That the training of physicians give increasing emphasis to the teaching of health and the prevention of disease, that adequate training be provided for nurse-midwives, that opportunities be offered for the systematic training of hospital and clinic administrators, etc.[2]

Timely as they may sound, these words were written more than a generation ago—in 1932—by the Committee on the Costs of Medical Care.

Today, we, as a nation, are facing essentially the same challenge that we faced more than a century ago. Is this because we are not adequately planning for changes to solve our health problems? Is it because our health planning techniques have not been used successfully? Or could it be that the products of the planning process have not been implemented?

The internal organization for planning has been discussed, but not the larger framework in which planning per se is effected, that is, external planning organizations.

EXTERNAL PLANNING ORGANIZATIONS IN HEALTH

The planning process can be carried out at national, regional, state, and local levels; furthermore, at these diverse levels, it can be accomplished through voluntary efforts or through governmental activities.

At the national level, health planning is a fragmented operation, with its activities spread among various agencies—both within and outside of the Federal Government. For the most part, therefore, it is not goal directed, since there are no coordinated, long-range, national health goals of a general policy nature.

Health planning at the regional level is complicated by the fact that, although the problems are local and the local point of view is the rationale

---

2 Committee on the Costs of Medical Care. *Medical Care for the American People*. Chicago, University of Chicago Press, 1933. pp. 103–144. Reprinted by Department of Health, Education, and Welfare, Washington, D.C., 1970.

behind planning, the solutions of today's health problems are regional. Since regions, however, involve more than one geopolitical entity, they lack the overall authority and the comprehensive expertise to plan and to implement planning at a regional level.

At the state level, we now have a comprehensive health planning agency in each state government. At the level of the governor's office, such an agency could overcome fragmentation; but, if placed at a lower level in the state government, such as in the health department, then the comprehensive health planning agency tends to become more parochial and limited in scope. This does not mean that the health department, as well as other agencies and organizations in the health field, should not maintain an internal organization for planning. The comprehensive health planning agency, however, should serve as the overall coordinating agency for long-range health planning.

In many ways, health planning at the local level has been an ongoing operation for years. The "1400 Governments Syndrome," exemplified by a study of the New York City metropolitan area, is a description of local government fragmentation. The average metropolitan area surely does not have 1,400 political subdivisions, but the ratio of political entities to population and area is probably similar. Planning at the local level, then, can be as fragmented and uncoordinated as health service is at this level.[3]

VOLUNTARY EFFORTS

Health planning in the United States has been accomplished through private efforts and at the official (governmental) level. Until very recently, however, voluntary efforts—that is, those of private or nongovernmental organizations —have predominated. Usually, these groups employed categorical approaches to the control of specific diseases. In recent years, governmental agencies too have participated in health planning activities. Similarly, their approach has been disease oriented and, in general, has been decentralized to the state or local levels. To illustrate this point, at the turn of the century, tuberculosis was recognized as a major national health problem by organized groups of voluntary health workers. Their efforts resulted in the establishment of programs for the prevention and treatment of tuberculosis in state and local public health agencies. Later, the National Tuberculosis Association extended its responsibilities and leadership and became the National Tuberculosis and Respiratory Disease Association; it will become the Amer-

3 Wood, Robert C. *1400 Governments Syndrome.* Cambridge, Mass., Harvard University Press, 1961.

ican Lung Association in the near future. This is one example, but similar patterns of health planning and program development have been followed for a variety of diseases by other large and well-known voluntary health agencies, such as the American Heart Association, the American Cancer Society, and others. These large, national, voluntary agencies—all with numerous local affiliates—communicate and coordinate their activities through the National Health Council.[4]

Historically, planning for health manpower was done on a voluntary basis and, at the outset, was stimulated by a study of medical education in the United States and Canada conducted by Abraham Flexner, who reported his findings in 1910. The Flexner report[5] advocated that medical care must be based on thorough knowledge of the biomedical sciences, that only high-quality medical schools should receive accreditation, that these schools should emphasize both laboratory work and intensive clinical experience, that many inadequate proprietary medical schools flourishing in that period should be closed down, and that medical schools should be affiliated with universities. As a result of these findings, the Flexner report led to pronounced changes over the subsequent 60 years in both medical education and the quality of medical care.

Fortunately, however, it has been recognized that, in planning for health manpower in modern times, the Flexner or research model has two weaknesses: first, it largely ignores health care delivery outside the medical school and the teaching hospital; and, second, it sets science in the medical school apart from science on the general campus, which results in duplication of effort. To offset these weaknesses, two new models appear to be arising: the health care delivery model and the integrated science model. These and other problems are being studied by the Carnegie Commission on Higher Education. A preliminary report by this Commission, titled *Higher Education and the Nation's Health—Policies for Medical and Dental Education*,[6] was issued in October 1970, and the final report was scheduled for completion in 1972.

An effort to resolve the problems resulting from rising costs and unequal distribution of medical care before and during the depression years was made

4 Stebbins, Ernest L. and Williams, Kathleen N. "History and Background of Health Planning in the United States." In: Reinke, W.A. *Health Planning: Qualitative Aspects and Quantitative Techniques.* Baltimore, Waverly Press, Inc., 1972. pp. 3–4.
5 Flexner, Abraham. *Medical Education in the United States and Canada.* New York, The Carnegie Foundation for the Advancement of Teaching, 1910.
6 Carnegie Commission on Higher Education. *Higher Education and the Nation's Health—Policies for Medical and Dental Education.* New York, McGraw-Hill, 1970.

by the Committee on the Costs of Medical Care. The recommendations of this Committee were discussed earlier (see pages 7 and 8).

Toward the end of World War II, the American Public Health Association and the National Health Council conducted a joint study on the provision of full-time, local health services in the United States.[7] The study examined traditional public health services (environmental sanitation, communicable disease control, maternal and child health, vital statistics, health education, and public health laboratory services) and set minimal standards for full-time, local health services based upon a very limited scope of program activity. These minimal standards became inadequate at a very early date because the field of public health and its responsibilities expanded so rapidly.

The problems of the aged and the chronically ill were brought to the attention of the public by the Commission on Chronic Illness, which was established under the auspices of the American Medical Association, the American Public Health Association, and the American Hospital Association. The four-volume report[8] issued by the Commission in the 1950's contributed a great deal to existing knowledge on the problems of finding and caring for the chronically ill. The impact of its recommendations, however, has not been fully realized.

A very recent, voluntarily supported, national planning effort, sponsored by the American Public Health Association and the National Health Council, was undertaken by the National Commission on Community Health Services.[9] The project was financed by foundation funds as well as by the U.S. Public Health Service and the Vocational Rehabilitation Administration. The Commission—representing health professionals, organized labor, industry, and the community at large—made a study of community health needs and existing services in order to develop a plan for a system of preventive and curative medical and environmental health services for the next decade. The report, published in the late 1960's, was a compilation of a series of monographs covering practically every phase of community health services. Many of its recommendations have now been implemented. Significantly, the Com-

---

[7] American Public Health Association, Committee on Administrative Practice, Subcommittee on Local Health Units. *Local Health Units for the Nation.* (Emerson Report) New York, The Commonwealth Fund, 1945.
[8] Commission on Chronic Illness. *Chronic Illness in the United States.* Vols. 1–4. Cambridge, Mass., Harvard University Press, 1956–1959.
[9] National Commission on Community Health Services. *Reports of the Task Forces on Environmental Health, Comprehensive Health Service, Health Manpower, Health Care Facilities, Financing of Health Services, Organization of Community Health Services.* Washington, D.C., Public Affairs Press, 1967.

mission recommended greater federal participation in community health services; also, comprehensive health planning on a continuing basis. It was through the research activities of this Commission that certain fundamentals relating to the planning process evolved. These included the concept of high-quality health care and a healthful environment as a civic right, the definition of a community of solution, and the recommendation of a single system for health care delivery rather than a fragmented public and private approach.[10,11]

GOVERNMENTAL HEALTH PLANNING

The Federal Government, through the Social Security Act of 1935, required states to develop plans for the control of specific diseases or, when this was not feasible, grants were provided to the states for the development of categorical programs for various specific purposes. These grants, usually made to the state health departments, resulted in the development of programs for maternal and child health care, tuberculosis and venereal disease control, services to crippled children, and, more recently, services in the various chronic disease categories such as heart disease, stroke, and cancer. The intent of this action was to stimulate program planning by the states and local communities; but, the fact that these grants were categorical and highly specific, eventually resulted in fragmentation, not only of these services, but also of the planning process at state and local levels.

Subsequent additional legislation has required planning for specific purposes at state and local levels. This legislation includes the Hospital Survey and Construction Act of 1946, the Heart, Cancer and Stroke Act of 1965, the Comprehensive Health Planning Act of 1966, and others, which are discussed later in this chapter.

COMMISSIONS

Several presidential commissions have influenced governmental health planning. In 1951, the President appointed the Commission on Health Needs of the Nation,[12] which represented professionals as well as consumers, particu-

---

10 National Commission on Community Health Services, Community Action Studies Project. *A Self-Study Guide for Community Action Planning.* New York, American Public Health Association, 1967.
11 National Commission on Community Health Services. *Health Is a Community Affair.* Cambridge, Mass., Harvard University Press, 1966.
12 President's Commission on the Health Needs of the Nation. *Building America's Health.* (Magnuson Report) Vols. 1–5. Washington, D.C., U.S. Government Printing Office, 1952–1953.

larly in labor and industry. The Commission studied the availability and adequacy of health services, facilities, and manpower and explored health needs and the extent to which the needs were being met, including in its study consumer opinions on the adequacy of programs and services. The Commission's report clearly identified the deficiencies and recommended major federal participation in financing more adequate services and facilities. The report, however, had little impact on the next administration or the Congress.[13]

A more influential presidential commission—the Commission on Heart Disease, Cancer and Stroke[14]—was established in 1963 for the purpose of identifying methods of reducing the toll taken by these diseases, particularly through better and faster utilization of existing medical knowledge. In less than a year, the Commission explored the morbidity and mortality problems of these several diseases and recommended, among other things, the establishment of a nationwide network of regional medical programs. The recommendations were enacted into law—though not exactly as the Commission had intended—with almost unheard of dispatch, and the Regional Medical Program Service began.

LEGISLATION, REGULATIONS, COMMITTEES

Specific committees of the U.S. Senate and House of Representatives deal with legislation and appropriations. Some of the current committees that deliberate on health matters are the Senate Finance Committee, the Senate Labor and Public Welfare Committee and its Subcommittee on Health, the Senate Appropriations Subcommittee on Labor and Health, the Senate Judiciary Subcommittee on Antitrust and Monopoly, the Senate Government Operations Subcommittee on Executive Reorganization, the House Ways and Means Committee, the House Interstate and Foreign Commerce Subcommittee on Public Health and Welfare, and the House Appropriations Subcommittee on Labor and Health.

The text for federal health laws can be found in the U.S. Code, Title 42; and there are federal regulations to assist in implementing these laws. Also available are numerous, specific documents on committee and congressional legis-

---

13 Stebbins, Ernest L. and Williams, Kathleen N. "History and Background of Health Planning in the United States." In: Reinke, W.A. *Health Planning: Qualitative Aspects and Quantitative Techniques.* Baltimore, Waverly Press, Inc., 1972. pp. 6–7.
14 President's Commission on Heart Disease, Cancer and Stroke. *A National Program to Conquer Heart Disease, Cancer and Stroke.* Washington, D.C., U.S. Government Printing Office, 1964.

lation. These are described in the handbook, *Legislative Research*, by Bergen and Reeves.[15]

REASONS FOR PLANNING

The idea of health planning is sensible and appealing. After all, health is considered a right—an inherent factor of social justice. Experienced health workers encourage planning; in fact, as a result of recent legislation, there is now some authority for planning. The economic benefits of planning are obvious, since planning is one way to get better value for every health dollar that is appropriated. The end result of health planning is, of course, to change things for the better by decreasing or resolving existing health problems in the United States. The less than optimum morbidity and mortality rates and the existence of preventable conditions such as malnutrition and polluted environment are clear indications that the United States, generically, does not have good health. Our health system is fraught with program gaps, and there are inconsistencies. It is worthwhile to mention, for example, that some programs are lacking, and that emphasis is on curative rather than preventive care; that there may be unequal distribution of resources, such as urban versus rural accessibility of services, not to mention intraurban or interurban differences; that fragmentation of services may occur, in which programs are neither interrelated nor working cooperatively, but, rather, are influenced by vested interests or solo practice; that in certain areas there may be a scarcity of health resources and suboptimal utilization of existing resources, resulting in increased demand and costs; and, finally, that there may exist the inability to make overall authoritative decisions for program implementation.

GOVERNMENTAL ACTION

Increasing governmental action in the health care field during recent years stems from widespread dissatisfaction with health services in the United States. Historically, medicine has followed a laissez-faire concept, and this

15 Bergen, K.M. and Reeves, P.N. *Legislative Research*. Washington, D.C., The George Washington University, 1971.

has made the planning process a difficult one. For example, planning cannot be undertaken without the cooperation of physicians, and it may meet outright opposition at the level of the American Medical Association. Even voluntary associations, that operate as areawide planning agencies on a private, nonprofit basis, have been unsuccessful, and they have not allayed consumer dissatisfaction.

Two alternatives appear to be available to the government: stimulation or coercion. At first, the government opted for stimulation via the grant-in-aid program; later, it moved toward coercion via legislation and regulation.

The grant-in-aid program, the development of federal health legislation, and current health planning programs are discussed in turn.

GRANTS-IN-AID

The federal grant-in-aid is a fiscal technique used to augment revenues of less affluent areas through legal transfer of funds accumulated by wealthier areas. The funds are redistributed on a formula basis dependent upon population characteristics, health problems (morbidity and mortality), and financial needs. Also, the recipient area often must produce the required matching funds, which can range from one-third to two-thirds of the total budget.

The grant-in-aid mechanism is a potent factor encouraging centralization consistent with the concept of federalism. Federal aid to states has been part of the U.S. scheme since early in its history and has included such things as development of militia (1808), land-grant colleges (beginning in the 1860's), public health funds for the control of venereal diseases (beginning in 1918), and other categorical grants. The grant-in-aid mechanism was used more frequently during the depression years, when state and local governments either could not or would not fund health programs. There have been some attempts in the past, notably during the Eisenhower Administration, to reverse this trend, without success; however, it appears that in the second term of the Nixon Administration such an effort will again be made. More than one health worker has recognized that many consider accepting funds from the government to be some sort of sinful alliance, but few are seen practicing abstinence.

PURPOSE

The grant-in-aid programs serve the following purposes:

1. *Equalize availability of programs.* By redistributing revenues, the grant-in-aid program fosters uniform availability of its programs throughout the nation, thus removing financial reasons for failure to develop a program.

2. *Stimulate program development and continuation.* The availability of categorical grant-in-aid funds—that is, funds specifically earmarked for a disease control program—made possible the development of programs for the control of tuberculosis, venereal diseases, heart diseases, cancer, and air pollution, as well as mental health programs, maternal and child health services, and radiological health programs. In the broad spectrum covered by grants-in-aid, there even exists a general health category that can be used for general programs such as multiphasic screening.

3. *Support a program of specific interest to the grantor.* In those instances where the grantor (namely, the Federal Government) had a specific interest, and the locality may or may not have had an interest, a grant-in-aid program was developed with the intent that local support would be afforded as the need for the program was demonstrated. An example of such a program might be one in which services to the aged would be developed.

4. *Supervise and control.* By stimulation with available funds, it is possible to avoid failures or program gaps due to local prejudice.

5. *Enforce minimum standards.* For example, in order to utilize grant-in-aid funds, health personnel to be employed by the program are required to meet certain qualifications.

6. *Distribute tax proceeds efficiently.* Since local and state governments are not as adept at tax collections as the Federal Government is, it was considered more efficient to use the federal collection agency for this purpose.

MECHANISM

The grant-in-aid program is more than just a donation of funds to the states by the Federal Government. In order to receive these funds, states are required to meet certain conditions: the state or locality to receive the funds must produce its proportionate share of matching funds; formal acceptance is required at the state level, sometimes necessitating legislative approval; a state plan describing the purpose, objectives, methodology, and evaluation of the program to be supported by these funds must be developed and must be approved by the Federal Government; the state must assure that it conforms to federal guidelines for such things as program recordkeeping, personnel qualifications, and program procedures; the state must agree to report data in an acceptable format; the state must provide periodic progress reports; and the state must submit to periodic fiscal auditing.

PROBLEMS

The federal grant-in-aid program has not been free of problems, some created by the program structure itself.

Of national concern is the varying degree of control among the states for any particular program.

The state and local problems have been many. The grant-in-aid program, being categorical—that is, distributing funds for specific program entities—has resulted in fragmentation of health activities at these levels. For the most part, specific programs are planned and carried out independently, without serious and effectual coordination with other programs. Thus, the maternal and child health program usually is entirely separate from the tuberculosis control, venereal disease, or general health programs. Further, federal priorities are foisted upon states without consideration for state and local priorities. This means that, from time to time, the state is forced to forego implementing a program which it considers of high priority because neither state nor federal funds are available for that category; federal grant-in-aid funds cannot be used for any category except the one for which the funds are appropriated. States also are uncertain as to whether specific grant-in-aid programs will continue to be funded. Continuation of funding is decided by the Federal Government on a year-to-year basis, with no guarantee that funds will continue beyond the current year, although, in fact, many grants are continued for many years. Such uncertainty makes it extremely difficult to hire and retain qualified personnel. Another financial problem is that the grant-in-aid program includes virtually no allowance for overhead costs, which often are not available at state or local levels. Frequently, in a grant-in-aid program, there is no provision for an increase in the total yearly allocation; this means that annual increments for salary or cost-of-living rises must be met either from local funds or by reducing the volume of the program in order to realize dollar savings which then can be applied toward increased costs. There also is a problem with the formula, which is not entirely equitable, since most plans result in proportionately more aid being granted to relatively better-off communities. Finally, states complain that the plan they are required to submit for approval in order to obtain grant-in-aid funds must cover not only the specific program to be supported by those funds, but also the entire health program of the state.

To sum up the problems concomitant with the federal grant-in-aid program, it appears that the most serious are fostering of fragmentation by the development of categorical programs, insufficient and uncertain funding, and lack of consideration for state and local priorities.

On the other hand, the new trend in federalism today is to place greater emphasis on regional and local decision making, thus providing more leeway for goal and priority determinations at state and local levels.

It should not be minimized or forgotten, however, that over the years the federal grant-in-aid program has resulted, in all states, in the development and continuation of programs to control tuberculosis and venereal diseases, to provide maternal and infant care, and to perform other services that otherwise might not have been uniformly available and might not have met acceptable standards.

The development of specific health planning legislation at the federal level began with the Hospital and Survey Construction Act (P.L. 79–725) passed by the U.S. Congress in 1946 and popularly known as the Hill-Burton program. In the several decades prior to the passage of the Hill-Burton Act and subsequent legislation, health program development followed two separate paths: the public sector of the health system, dealing with the role of government in the provision of health services; and the private sector of the health system, including practitioners and hospitals, which did some planning on an areawide basis, principally for the development of facilities such as hospitals.

HILL-BURTON ACT

The Hospital Survey and Construction Act, P.L. 79–725, was passed in August 1946. It comprises Title VI of the Public Health Service Act and provides for the Hill-Burton program.

HISTORY

By 1946, there was a general shortage of hospital beds in the nation; more than one-third of the counties had *no* hospital beds. Not only were they unevenly distributed geographically, but, in addition, there was little coordination among them. This condition existed because few new hospitals had been constructed during the depression years of the 1930's and the years of restrictions imposed by World War II; furthermore, existing facilities had become obsolete. The problem was compounded by rapid population growth, migration from rural to urban areas, and rapidly rising construction costs. Along with the shortage of beds, especially in rural areas, there was a shortage of medical personnel.

A number of proposals were made calling for government action in the hospital field. It took several years, however, to get such legislation enacted by Congress because, in the aftermath of World War II, the Administration was preoccupied with foreign affairs rather than with domestic problems and because physicians and hospital associations were critical of proposed legislation and ignored the financial plight of the voluntary hospital.

Once passed, however, the program continued at an accelerating pace and, through the years, was expanded by amendments.

PROVISIONS

In its initial form, the 1946 Hill-Burton Act authorized grants to states for the purpose of:

1. Surveying their needs; developing plans for the construction of facilities, including public and other nonprofit hospitals; and establishing adequate hospitals, clinics, and similar services for all the people.
2. Assisting in the construction and equipment of needed public and voluntary nonprofit general, mental, tuberculosis, and chronic disease hospitals and public health centers.

The Act authorized the appropriation of a minimum allocation to each state according to population. The states could draw upon these allotments to meet up to one-third of the expenses necessary for carrying out the provisions of the Act. Each state was required to designate a single state agency and an advisory council to implement its program; also, to establish a plan for conducting a survey of existing hospitals and related facilities in order to develop a program for needed construction. The state agencies established one or more regions within state boundaries for planning purposes; however, the Hill-Burton Act and its amendments did nothing to encourage cooperation or regional coordination among health facilities, requiring only that there be a rational geographic distribution of beds.

In 1949, amendments to the Hill-Burton Act authorized the U.S. Public Health Service to provide grants for and conduct research, experiments, and demonstrations relating to the development, effective utilization, and coordination of hospital services, facilities, and resources. It took until 1956, however, before appropriations to carry out these amendments were provided.

Additional amendments in 1954 broadened the Hill-Burton program to include specific grants for construction of public and voluntary nonprofit nursing homes, diagnostic or treatment centers, rehabilitation facilities, and chronic disease facilities.

The 1958 amendments to the Hill-Burton Act gave sponsors that met standard eligibility and priority qualifications the option to take long-term loans in lieu of grants. In 1961, under the Community Health Services and Facilities Act, the annual appropriation authorized for construction of nurs-, ing homes was increased, as was the annual research appropriation for experimental and demonstration construction and equipment projects. It is of considerable importance to note that this latter Act also was used by the Federal Government to provide funds to planning agencies.

Amendments which extended the program through June 1969 were added to the Hospital Survey and Construction Act in 1964. Its title subsequently was changed to the Health and Medical Facilities Survey and Construction Act, and it is now known as the Hill-Harris Act (P.L. 91–296). The provisions included not only grants and loans for new construction, but also provided for modernization and replacement of all kinds of facilities. In addition, a program of project grants was authorized to develop comprehensive regional, metropolitan, or other local-area plans for health and related facilities (Section 318). Previously, demonstration grants supported areawide planning efforts; however, in June 1967, funding for comprehensive health planning agencies was transferred to the Comprehensive Health Planning Program. This program, authorized by the Partnership for Health Act, repealed the Hill-Burton Research and Demonstration Project grants and set up the National Center for Health Services Research and Development. This Act is discussed in greater detail in Chapter 2.

FUNCTION

The Hill-Burton Act designated a state agency and an advisory council and required an annually updated Hill-Burton Plan for Survey and Construction of Hospital and Related Facilities that would comply with standards.[16,17]

16 U.S. Department of Health, Education, and Welfare, Public Health Service, Division of Hospital and Medical Facilities, Program Planning and Analysis Branch. *Facts About the Hill-Burton Program*. Washington, D.C., U.S. Government Printing Office, 1968.
17 U.S. Department of Health, Education, and Welfare, Public Health Service, Division of Hospital and Medical Facilities, Program Planning and Analysis Branch. *Hill-Burton Is . . .* Washington, D.C., U.S. Government Printing Office, 1968.

PROBLEMS

The Hill-Burton program generated many small rural hospitals that were economically unsound, but did not influence the delivery system itself. It also did not result in coordination among hospitals or among hospitals and other health facilities, beyond what had already developed sporadically as a result of the private practice of medicine. The Act, of course, did not require this; but, on the other hand, there was no demand for it. Initially, the need for beds had been so great that the system under which the beds were provided was not important, and coordination of health facilities as a desirable end was not recognized beyond what already informally existed. By the late 1950's and the early 1960's, however, it was apparent that a regional system for interrelationships and coordination among health facilities was needed, but not necessarily with a medical center as its core. Thus evolved the concept of a partnership that would link government and voluntary agencies and that would involve the Hill-Burton program as one part of a total comprehensive health program. This resulted in P.L. 89–749, the Comprehensive Health Planning and Public Health Service Amendments Act of 1966.

ACCOMPLISHMENTS

The Hill-Burton program did achieve its purposes by reducing the wide range of bed-to-population ratios. Today, however, the value of such a ratio is questionable. The program also increased the total number of beds so that few areas have either an excess or a shortage; it modernized facilities to a lesser degree than it constructed new facilities; it encouraged the states to adopt and improve licensure laws; it reduced reliance upon philanthropy as a source of funds; and, since public funds now are involved, it created a sense of community responsibility for health facilities. In fact, it provided a good working example of cooperation among all levels of government while remaining attuned to local needs. The extension legislation for the Hill-Harris Program (P.L. 91–296, 1970) and for the Comprehensive Health Planning Program (P.L. 91–515, 1970) recognized the need to tie hospital and health facility construction planning more closely to the comprehensive health planning process.[18,19]

---

[18] U.S. Department of Health, Education, and Welfare, Health Services and Mental Health Administration, Health Facility Planning and Construction Service, Office of Program Planning and Analysis. *Hill-Burton Program Progress Report, July 1, 1947–June 30, 1969.* Washington, D.C., U.S. Government Printing Office, Revised 1969. PHS Publication No. 930–F–3.
[19] Reeves, Philip N. "Analysis of the Hill-Burton Program." Washington, D.C., The George Washington University, Department of Health Care Administration, 1967. Unpublished paper.

REFERENCES

1. American Hospital Association. *Statement on Planning*. Chicago, 1969. 551r.
2. "Free Care in Hill-Burton Hospitals." Editorial in *Modern Medicine*, August 7, 1972. p. 15.
3. Hanlon, John J. *Principles of Public Health Administration*. 5th Edition. Saint Louis, C.V. Mosby Co., 1969. pp. 130–136, 151–157.
4. "Hill-Burton Funding Would Be Changed." *Modern Medicine*, October 16, 1972. p. 21. Washington Report.
5. May, J. Joel. *Health Planning: Its Past and Potential*. Chicago, Center for Health Administration Studies, University of Chicago, 1967. pp. 13–45.
6. P.L. 79–725. *Hospital Survey and Construction Act* (Hill-Burton Program). Washington, D.C., U.S. Government Printing Office, 1946.
7. P.L. 88–443. *Hospital and Medical Facilities Amendments* (Hill-Harris Program). Washington, D.C., U.S. Government Printing Office, 1964.
8. Piel, Gerard. "Technological Change in the Medical Economy." In: *Planning for Health; Report of the 1967 Health Forum*. New York, National Health Council, 1968. pp. 188–197.
9. "Poor Demand More Hospital Care." *Modern Medicine,* January 8, 1973. p. 26.

CHAPTER 2

CURRENT PLANNING PROGRAMS

The preceding chapter discussed the history of health planning; why and how the government became involved in health planning; and the development of health planning legislation, including the grant-in-aid program, the Hill-Burton program, and recent amendments providing for areawide planning.

A number of laws currently provide for health and health-related planning, and the following five of these laws will be reviewed:

P.L. 88–164   The Mental Retardation Facilities and Community Mental Health Centers Act of 1963

P.L. 89–4   The Appalachian Regional Development Act of 1965 (amended by P.L. 90–103)

P.L. 89–239   The Heart, Cancer and Stroke Amendments of 1965 (known as the Regional Medical Program)

P.L. 89–749   The Comprehensive Health Planning and Public Health Service Amendments Acts of 1966 (known as the Partnership for Health Act)

P.L. 89–754   The Comprehensive City Demonstrations Program of 1966 (known as Model Cities Program)

THE MENTAL RETARDATION FACILITIES AND COMMUNITY HEALTH CENTERS ACT OF 1963

This legislation is the cornerstone for improvements in mental health services. It was fostered and promoted by the family of the late President John F. Kennedy.

PURPOSES AND PROVISIONS

In order to combat the ravages of mental retardation, this Act provides funds for the construction of research centers, as well as grants for the construction

23

of facilities to serve the mentally retarded. The Act also provides for the development of community mental health centers through grants for the construction, planning, and staffing of such centers. Subsequent amendments to the Act provide for facilities for alcoholics and drug addicts.

Each state is required to designate a single state agency and an advisory council to develop a state plan that must provide for the following five basic services: inpatient care, outpatient care, partial hospitalization, emergency care, and consultation and education.

The overall intent of this Act is to provide for the prevention of mental illness and for the care of the mentally ill at the community level by offering a continuing series of coordinated programs within the community. This is an alternative to the former approach, which institutionalized mentally ill patients in large mental hospitals away from the community.[1,2]

PROBLEMS

In general, this legislation has been successful in promoting community services, improved facilities, and increased knowledge about the care of the mentally ill and the retarded; however, the program has not been without its problems. There is some feeling that the target population (anywhere from 75,000 to 200,000 people) required for the establishment of a community mental health center is too large for a community program.

The Act provides for little flexibility or local option relative to the size of the facility and the target population. For example, if the "catchment area" concept was used, as encouraged, then the community mental health center would be depicted as being in the very vortex of the reservoir—with patients and clients coming to it for services—rather than as a decentralized program reaching out toward the periphery of the catchment area. There is some feeling at the state level that the National Institute of Mental Health, which has the responsibility for implementing this Act, superimposed its philosophy upon state and local advisory boards and programs rather than pursuing joint and cooperative planning with states and localities.

Further, the program is structured to provide for a decrease in funds yearly—over a period of five years—at which time the states must take over

1 Lemkau, Paul V. and Mandell, Wallace. "History and Special Features of Mental Health Planning." In: Reinke, W.A. *Health Planning: Qualitative Aspects and Quantitative Techniques.* Baltimore, Waverly Press, Inc., 1972. pp. 279–288.
2 U.S. Department of Health, Education, and Welfare, Health Services and Mental Health Administration, National Institute of Mental Health. *The Comprehensive Community Mental Health Centers Program.* Washington, D.C., U.S. Government Printing Office, 1969.

with other funds. The states are finding it difficult to provide local funds for such a large and complex program within the relatively short period of five years. The problem is compounded by the fact that the grants provide for professional staff salaries only, which means that the local areas must assume the responsibility for raising funds for nonprofessional and administrative staff salaries.

Finally, a longer range, programmatic problem faces the community; namely, that community mental health centers have developed independently from physical health programs. Therefore, there is a need to coordinate mental health programs with general health programs; they cannot be separated, since mental health is obviously one part of total health.

THE APPALACHIAN REGIONAL DEVELOPMENT ACT OF 1965

Although the Appalachian program is not specifically a health program, it has many provisions that affect health planning. Basically, in the overall concept, this Act provides for public works and economic development programs in the Appalachian Region of the United States. Interest in the Act, however, relates to two provisions which can be utilized in the area of health planning. In one instance, the Act provides for establishment of the Appalachian Regional Commission. This joint state and federal Commission is authorized to perform comprehensive planning and coordination, which can include the planning of health programs. There has been some controversy, however, over the relative power of the states versus the Federal Government in the functioning of the Regional Commission.[3,4] In the other instance, the Act provides for funding of demonstration health facilities through grants for construction, equipment, and operation of health facilities. Any agency or organization is eligible to apply for these funds.[5,6]

---

[3] Hearle, Edward. "The Regional Commissions: Approach to Economic Development." *Public Administration Review*, 28(1):17, January–February 1968.

[4] Hamilton, Randy. "The Regional Commissions: A Restrained View." *Public Administration Review*, 28(1):20–21, January–February 1968.

[5] U.S. Department of Health, Education, and Welfare, Health Services and Mental Health Administration, Office of Grants Management. *Profiles of Grant Programs, HSMHA.* 1971 Edition. Washington, D.C., U.S. Government Printing Office, 1971. pp. 3–8. Stock number 1720–0033.

[6] Office of Economic Opportunity. *Catalog of Federal Domestic Assistance.* Compiled by the Office of Management and Budget. Washington, D.C., U.S. Government Printing Office, 1970.

THE HEART, CANCER AND STROKE AMENDMENTS OF 1965

This legislation is the first significant attempt to organize health services along regional rather than geopolitical lines. It is a result of deliberations by the President's Commission on Heart Disease, Cancer and Stroke (the De Bakey Commission), appointed in 1964 to study these three major causes of death.

PURPOSES AND PROVISIONS

One of the purposes of this Act is to encourage and assist in the establishment of regional cooperative arrangements among medical schools, research institutions, and hospitals in order to conduct research, provide training and continuing education, and carry out demonstrations of patient care. It is the further intent of the Act that such arrangements will serve to create greater opportunities for making available to patients the latest advances in the diagnosis and treatment of heart disease, cancer, stroke, kidney, and related diseases, thus improving generally the health services, manpower, and facilities available to the nation.

The Heart, Cancer and Stroke Amendments of 1965 resulted in the creation of 56 regions—encompassing all 50 states and territorial possessions in the United States—with each setting up its own Regional Medical Program (RMP). The program design for each region is determined locally, and the scope and nature of services are subject to the decision of the local planning body (known as the Regional Advisory Group). The initial general strategy for the various RMPs was to organize existing provider resources into cooperative arrangements aimed at improving health care in the specific disease categories covered by this legislation and, later, to include kidney disease. Experience, legislative modification, and administrative interpretation have produced substantial evolutionary changes in the Regional Medical Program so that the basic disease-oriented thrust has now been diminished. In its place, top priority consideration is being given to the availability and accessibility of quality health care. Furthermore, emphasis is now being placed upon outpatient and ambulatory services rather than upon institutionally based services at hospitals or medical centers; also, more emphasis is being placed upon prevention of disease rather than solely upon treatment or curative services.[7,8]

The Regional Medical Program deals not only with medical centers, hospitals, and related facilities, but also with practicing physicians; therefore, it may be described as the only link between the Federal Government and the private sector of medicine.

The RMP is indeed very important to the delivery of health services along regional lines, but it should also be examined in the light of the problems and controversies that it faces.

PROBLEMS AND ISSUES

There has been much speculation on the future of this program. Many of the Regional Medical Programs have been successful in combining elements of the health care delivery systems that previously were isolated and independent of each other. Others have promoted the extension of new medical knowledge from the medical centers into the offices of private practitioners and community hospitals. Yet, the recent changes in emphasis have created confusion about the program's mission and the means to achieve that mission. One particular problem that must be considered is whether the role of Regional Medical Programs is to change—rather than simply upgrade—the existing health care delivery system. This type of role seems threatening to the providers of health care.

Another problem involves the relationship of the Regional Medical Program to the Comprehensive Health Planning (CHP) Program. Is there sufficient justification for two separate programs: one dealing primarily with providers and with the chronic diseases previously mentioned; the other dealing primarily with consumers on a more comprehensive basis, but not necessarily on a regional basis.[9]

There is also some concern about the responsibility of the Regional Medical Program for regionalization. Health providers apparently oppose a highly structured regional system in which the patient flow would be from the periphery to the center, whereas manpower and services would flow from the

[7] Weinerman, F.R. "The Regional Concept," from "Regionalization of Medical Services." In: Committee on Medical Care Teaching. *Readings in Medical Care.* Chapel Hill, N.C., University of North Carolina Press, 1958. pp. 350–356. (First published in 1949.)
[8] Regional Medical Programs Service. *Progress Report.* Washington, D.C., U.S. Government Printing Office, 1970. (#404–181)
[9] Bryan, James E. "View from the Hill." *American Family Physician,* 4(2):125–127, August 1971.

center toward the periphery. As far as the public is concerned, however, it appears that their major concerns are accessibility and cost of health care; regionalization, although obviously relevant, is not yet a public issue. The Regional Medical Program does not have legislated responsibility for accomplishing regionalization; nevertheless, its mission is to develop regional cooperative arrangements as voluntary efforts to bring together isolated elements of the health system. These linkages, of course, should be used as a means of achieving improved health care and should not be used as an end in themselves. Another issue is that the future of the RMP must be considered in relation to its present limitations, which include funding restrictions, confusion in Washington over the federal health policy and relationships between similar federal programs, less than full cooperation from organized medicine, and "town-gown rivalries." Nevertheless, the RMP appears to be at a crossroads. Certainly, this is the organization that is taking some steps toward regionalization, that is bringing increased attention to continuing medical education, and that is demonstrating the growing governmental belief of decentralizing authority in favor of local agencies. It has moved from a more categorical, institutionally based program toward a more comprehensive program for the delivery of health care services.[10,11,12]

THE COMPREHENSIVE HEALTH PLANNING AND PUBLIC HEALTH SERVICE AMENDMENTS ACT OF 1966

P.L. 89–749 was enacted in 1966, essentially to integrate the various health activities that the health care delivery system had been developing on an ad hoc basis. Planning agencies could rely only on persuasion and education. There had been large increases in the number of health programs and activities, in the volume of funds being spent within the health care industry, and in the number of both official and unofficial groups involved in planning and service. Pressure had built up across the nation for legal authority and enforceable sanctions, control of financial resources, control of quality through

[10] Bodenheimer, Thomas S., M.D. "RMPs: No Road to Regionalization." *Medical Care Review,* 26(11):1125–1166, December 1969.
[11] Page, Irvin H., M.D. "Are Regional Medical Programs Worth It?" *Modern Medicine,* August 9, 1971. pp. 61–66.
[12] Komaroff, Anthony L., M.D. "Regional Medical Programs in Search of a Mission." *New England Journal of Medicine,* 284(14):758–764, April 8, 1971.

licensing, and even for a federal regulatory agency that would regulate the health care system as if it were a public utility. The result of all this ferment was the development of the "partnership for health" or "umbrella" concept embodied in the Comprehensive Health Planning and Public Health Service Amendments Act of 1966, namely, to correct fragmentation; to link all planning and all services—public, private, or voluntary—into a cooperative, coordinated approach; and to include not only personal health services, but environmental health services and facilities and manpower as well.

The Congress declared that, "The fulfillment of our national purpose depends upon promoting and assuring the highest level of health attainable, for every person, in an environment which contributes positively to healthful, individual and family living," and then found that comprehensive planning for health services, health manpower, and health facilities would be essential for carrying out that purpose.

Comprehensive health planning is a continuous process through which both providers and consumers can arrive at an agreement regarding health needs, goals, and priorities; resources and measures appropriate to the achievement of goals; and recommendations for action by public and private sectors to enhance the effectiveness of existing resources and activities and to develop those needed for the future. Comprehensive health planning differs from functional or specialized health planning in that it focuses on the total health needs of all people, rather than only on those related to a specific problem, such as mental illness; on a particular type of service, such as restaurant sanitation; or on a specific population group, such as children. Comprehensive health planning, however, does not diminish the need for specialized health planning or for specific program planning by operating health agencies. It should provide, instead, the framework within which planning for specialized functions and for special programs can be related to the state and community priorities and objectives agreed upon.

PROVISIONS

The most significant provisions are contained in Sections 314(a) through (e), descriptions of which follow:

Section 314(a) – Formula Grants to States for Comprehensive Health Planning: Each state must designate a single state agency to administer the planning function and to develop a plan for comprehensive health planning, which must be approved by the Secretary of Health, Education, and Welfare.

This agency can be located in the office of the governor, in the state health department, or it can be an interdepartmental agency or board.

The state plan for comprehensive health planning must provide for the establishment of a state health planning council, to include representatives from state and local agencies, nongovernmental organizations, health practitioners, and other groups concerned with health. A majority of this council must represent consumers of health services. Consumers are defined as those persons who do not work in the health field.

All 50 of the eligible states and territorial governments have received approval of their state plans and are funded to organize and conduct statewide comprehensive health planning. The 314(a) funds are allocated on the basis of population and per capita income.

Section 314(b) – Project Grants for Areawide Comprehensive Health Planning: Public or private nonprofit agencies or organizations may apply for grants to develop comprehensive regional or local health planning in coordination with existing and planned health services, manpower, and facilities. Applications must be approved by the state health planning agency to assure coordination of local and state health planning efforts. Most of the sponsoring agencies are voluntary nonprofit organizations, some are local governments, and others are local councils of government. Geographically, project areas are not confined to a single county or state, but can range in size from single counties to several counties in two or more states.

Grantees are required to establish advisory health planning councils composed of representatives of providers and consumers of health services, with a majority of the membership consisting of consumers. If the areawide planning agency is not a part of the local government, then it must provide for representation from the local government.

Section 314(c) – Project Grants for Training, Studies, and Demonstrations in Health Planning: Grants to improve health planning skills and knowledge may be awarded to public or private nonprofit agencies, institutions, or organizations, including universities. Primary emphasis is on training people in planning skills. Grants may support graduate education, continuing education, and training of consumers for participation in comprehensive health planning.

Section 314(d) – Formula Grants to State Health Authorities and Mental Health Authorities for Public Health Services: Grants under this Section are awarded to help establish and maintain a full range of public health services. These funds are not restricted for use in meeting specific disease problems, but rather are meant primarily to provide the states with the opportunity to initiate new and different methods of furnishing health protection. The objective is to innovate where innovation is needed, particularly when such important health services cannot be supported with existing state or local funds. The provisions of this Section are considered to be a single block grant which replaces the former 15 categorical formula grants.

A plan for the provision of public health and mental health services is required from each state. This plan is to be developed by the state health and mental health departments and must be compatible with the total comprehensive health plan of the state.

The amount of each grant is based on a state's population and its per capita income. States must allocate at least 15 percent of their block grant funds to the mental health authority and must provide at least 70 percent of their total grant funds for health services at the community level, rather than use these funds for state-level administrative costs. The manner in which each state allocates its grant funds is closely followed, with up to 1 percent of the appropriations under this Section being made available to the Department of Health, Education, and Welfare (HEW) for evaluation of these public health services.

The grants under this Section are allocated to state health agencies which, in turn, re-allocate the funds to appropriate community agencies.

Section 314(e) – Project Grants for Health Services Development: Priority for grants under this Section of the Comprehensive Health Planning Program is given to those projects, especially in disadvantaged communities, that are designed to deliver comprehensive health services that focus on programs of organized primary care. In other words, these funds are allocated on a project grant basis to meet specific limited needs or to develop new methods of health care delivery. Innovation in the delivery of such services is encouraged, and new or improved health care systems that increase efficiency and reduce costs are supported whenever possible. Active consumer and provider participation in the development and operation of comprehensive health service projects is sought. Any public or private nonprofit agency can apply for a project grant to be used for health services development.

In keeping with the intent of the legislation, health services supported by grants under this Section must be provided in accordance with the state comprehensive health plan. Applications for grants under this Section also must be referred to the appropriate areawide health planning agencies for review and comment; however, if such agencies do not exist, then applications must be reviewed by other public or private nonprofit agencies performing similar functions.

Again, up to 1 percent of the total grants awarded under this part of the program must be made available to HEW for evaluation of these health services development projects.

This completes the review of Sections 314(a) through (e) of The Comprehensive Health Planning and Public Health Service Amendments Act of 1966 (Partnership for Health Act). Following is a discussion of how programs under this Act operate and what is being done to implement them as prescribed by these laws.

IMPLEMENTATION AND FUNCTIONS
The Partnership for Health program was amended by P.L. 90–174 and P.L. 91–515. These amendments strengthened the program by increasing and extending its funding authorizations and by requiring the establishment of a national advisory council on comprehensive health planning programs, with council membership to be representative of consumers as well as providers of health services. The Partnership for Health program is administered by the Community Health Service of the Health Services Administration (HSA) of HEW. This program represents a concerted effort on the part of the Federal Government to consolidate a large number of parallel programs operating at state and local levels, thereby eliminating duplication of services and improving efficiency. With amendments, this program gives the states greater flexibility in supporting comprehensive health services by allowing them to channel grant funds into those programs for which there is the greatest need. The comprehensive health planning agency is an advocate of the public interest in health and provides the mechanisms for consumer input into health planning. It further provides the setting and means for tripartite participation in rational decision making; that is, involvement by the consumer, the provider, and the government. Its responsibilities, however, do not end when plans and recommenda-

tions are made, but continue until they are carried out and the results are evaluated in terms of intended accomplishments.[13,14,15,16,17]

ISSUES AND PROBLEMS

One issue of considerable interest is the relationship between the 314(a) and (b) agencies and, in turn, the relationship of these agencies to the Regional Medical Program.

The relationship between state- and area-level comprehensive health planning agencies depends upon similarities and differences in their functions and upon authority vested in them to carry out these functions.

On the one hand, comprehensive health planning at the area and state levels is similar, in that it focuses on all the people and all their needs. Its processes are similar in concept at both levels—although they may vary in detail—and include such things as data gathering, goal setting, development of alternatives, review or approval of government grants and government-supported programs, and may even encompass licensure of hospitals and extended care facilities.

On the other hand, the difference between the two levels lies chiefly in the subjects that are dealt with in planning recommendations and decisions. At the state level, in most states, these are chiefly matters of broad policy affecting the entire state or whole groups of institutions, activities, or resources. At the area level, these planning procedures and decisions are more often specific to particular institutions, activities, or resources.

The 314(a) agency must approve plans for the establishment of a 314(b) agency before it can be set up. The 314(a) and (b) agencies then share data and information and coordinate planning, recruitment, and training.

What is the source of influence, or what authority does the comprehensive health planning agency have? Certainly, the legislation goes far to encourage

---

13 Roseman, Cyril. "Problems and Prospects for CHP." *American Journal of Public Health,* *62*(1):16–19, January 1972.
14 U.S. Department of Health, Education, and Welfare. *Comprehensive Health Planning, Comprehensive Health Services Fact Sheet.* Washington, D.C., U.S. Government Printing Office, 1971. (#420–928)
15 U.S. Department of Health, Education, and Welfare. *Comprehensive Health Planning.* Washington, D.C., U.S. Government Printing Office, 1971. (#418–782)
16 U.S. Department of Health, Education, and Welfare, Public Health Service, Health Services and Mental Health Administration, Community Health Service, Division of Comprehensive Health Planning. *1971–1972 Graduate Education in Comprehensive Health Planning.* Washington, D.C., U.S. Government Printing Office, 1971. Publication No. HSM–71–6103.
17 Community Health, Inc. "Legislation—New Programs, New Philosophies." *Health Planning Issue Paper #1.* New York, March 1970.

—indeed to provide—a mandate for comprehensive health planning by providing funds and establishing a structure for its implementation. The influence of the comprehensive health planning agency arises to a considerable extent from its continuing function of providing the means and setting for participation by all interested parties. The areawide comprehensive health planning agency has been given certain responsibilities for review and comment on applications for federally financed projects. Beyond this, there is no overall authority delegated to the state or areawide planning agencies. It is interesting to note that a few states have attempted to establish and define the legal authority of their 314(a) and (b) agencies through the delegation of responsibility for licensure of hospitals and nursing homes and through the regulation of rates.

A good planning process does not necessarily, in and of itself, result in the improvement of health care. Actually, the Partnership for Health legislation does not really touch upon many of the obstacles that have hampered implementation of past planning decisions, such as unenlightened self-interest, parochialism, and vaguely defined objectives.

The role of the consumer—and how it is to be played—is still another issue in the comprehensive health planning program. How is a truly representative consumer elected or selected? How does that consumer avoid being co-opted by the program when he becomes a functionary within it? Is the consumer's role a controlling one, an advisory one, or some combination of the two?

The formula or block grant provided under Section 314(d) also has its problems; for instance, the total block allocation has increased very little over the total funding that previously was provided by the various categorical grants. If previous funding is obligated to existing programs which cannot be reduced or eliminated, then, in effect, there is no advantage to combining all of these programs into a single block grant. Furthermore, special-interest groups complain about the block grant because, by including their specific program with others, they feel they have lost the visibility of being identified as a categorical program.

With reference to the special-project grants authorized under Section 314(e), the problem here seems to be one of competition, since each applicant for these funds must compete with all other applicants in a region of the United States and is not subject to decentralized decision making or to the provisions of the state plan. Also, there is concern about underfunding of Section 314(e).

The role of the Federal Government in the Partnership for Health program has not been clarified. Is its role to be simply one of horizontal coordination, or should it be one of total involvement? Should comprehensive health planning be accomplished at all levels—federal, state, and local—as well as within HEW and between HEW and other departments involved with health matters, such as OEO, Labor, Justice, HUD, Defense, and others?

It has been discouraging to health planners and health workers that the comprehensive health planning program at state and local levels has developed at such a very slow pace and, in many places, has not yet reached maturity. Many agencies are still performing essentially a review and comment function rather than actually practicing comprehensive health planning. Also, some feeling exists that there is relative underemphasis on environmental health services when compared to personal health services.

In order to relate the position of comprehensive health planning agencies to other government planning programs, more understanding of their functions is needed. For example, the relationship between the Hill-Burton state agency and the state and areawide comprehensive health planning agencies is still being clarified, as is the relationship of the CHP agencies to the Regional Medical Program, the Model Cities Program, the Council of Governments, and other planning or coordinating groups. It is becoming clearer that comprehensive health planning builds upon the specialized planning of Regional Medical Programs, Hill-Burton programs, and others, but, in actual accomplishment, does not replace them. Comprehensive health planning agencies coordinate all these programs, utilize their data, and keep them informed. A scarcity of professional health planners is a common problem.[18,19,20,21,22,23]

18 Robins, Leonard. "The Impact of Decategorizing Federal Programs—Before and After 314(d)." *American Journal of Public Health*, 62(1):24–29, January 1972.

19 U.S. Department of Health, Education, and Welfare, Health Services and Mental Health Administration, Community Health Service, Division of Comprehensive Health Planning. *An Advocate of the Public Interest*. Washington, D.C., U.S. Government Printing Office, 1971. Publication No. HSM 71–6108.

20 U.S. Department of Health, Education, and Welfare, Public Health Service, Health Services and Mental Health Administration, Community Health Service, Division of Comprehensive Health Planning. *1971–1972 Graduate Education in Comprehensive Health Planning*. Washington, D.C., U.S. Government Printing Office, 1971. Publication No. HSM 71–6103.

21 Community Health, Inc. "Legislation—New Programs, New Philosophies." *Health Planning Issue Paper #1*. New York, March 1970.

22 Batistella, Roger M. "The Course of Regional Health Planning." *Medical Care*, 4:149–161, May–June 1967.

23 Anderson, Nancy N. *Comprehensive Health Planning in the States: A Study and Critical Analysis*. Minneapolis, Institute for Interdisciplinary Studies, American Rehabilitation Foundation, 1968. pp. 30–38.

THE COMPREHENSIVE CITY DEMONSTRATIONS PROGRAM OF 1966

The Comprehensive City Demonstrations Program (also known as the Model Cities Program) does not specifically legislate for health planning, but health planning is incorporated as one of its activities.

PROVISIONS AND PURPOSES

This Act provides grants and technical assistance for the rebuilding and restoration of slum and blighted areas in the nation's cities. It also provides for the establishment of a City Demonstrations Agency (CDA) and administers the Model Cities Program in a city or county. As stated in the Act, the CDA may be a city, county, or any local public agency established or designed by the local government that desires to have a Model Cities grant.

In addition to the CDA, there must be an elected Commission, as well as a state plan—updated annually—for the utilization of the Model Cities grant funds. The elected Commission must approve all plans and programs for the Model Cities area regardless of the source of funds.

The Comprehensive City Demonstrations Program is implemented by the Department of Housing and Urban Development at the federal level.[24]

This completes the review of the five laws providing for health and health-related planning that are pertinent to this discussion of current planning programs. The remainder of this chapter examines the extent to which federal agencies can cooperate with state and local governments in the implementation of the various federally sponsored assistance programs.

EVALUATION, REVIEW, AND COORDINATION OF FEDERAL AND FEDERALLY ASSISTED PROJECTS

Circular No. A-95 (Revised) of the Office of Management and Budget of the Executive Office of the President provides guidance to federal agencies on

[24] Office of Economic Opportunity. *Catalog of Federal Domestic Assistance.* Compiled by the Office of Management and Budget. Washington, D.C., U.S. Government Printing Office, 1970.

how to obtain added cooperation from state and local governments in the evaluation, review, and coordination of federal assistance programs and projects. This *Circular* promulgates the regulations for implementation of the provisions of Section 204 of the Demonstration Cities and Metropolitan Development Act of 1966 and of Title IV of the Intergovernmental Co-operation Act of 1968. These laws contain provisions for the following: establishing a project notification and review system to facilitate coordinated planning on an intergovernmental basis for several federal assistance programs; coordinating direct federal development programs and projects with state, regional, and local planning groups; and securing the comments and views of state and local agencies that are authorized to develop and enforce environmental standards.

OMB *Circular No. A-95* also sets up the following guidelines for federal agencies in their dealings with state, regional, and local governments: a project notification and review system; information about direct federal development and state plans; relationship information concerning state plans; and coordination of planning in multijurisdictional areas.

Project Notification and Review System: The project notification and review system requires that a network of state, regional, and metropolitan planning and development clearinghouses be established to aid in the coordination of federal or federally assisted projects and programs with state, regional, and local planning in order to stimulate orderly growth and development. Any agency of a state or local government, or any applicant for assistance under a federal program, will be required to notify the planning and development clearinghouse of the state and the region—if there is one—of its intent to apply for a federal grant and to provide the clearinghouse with a summary description of the proposed project. The clearinghouse will evaluate the significance of the proposal to state, areawide, or local plans, as appropriate; it will disseminate project notifications to the proper state and local agencies; it will provide whatever liaison may be necessary between such agencies and the applicant; and, finally, it will arrange to consult with the applicant—as often as necessary—on the proposed project. Comments and recommendations made by or through clearinghouses are for the purpose of assuring maximum consistency of a specific project with state, regional, and local comprehensive plans. These comments also are intended to assist the federal or state agency administering the program in determining whether it is in accord with applicable federal law.

Information About Direct Federal Development and State Plans: Circular No. A-95 stipulates that state and local governments be provided with information on projected federal developments to facilitate coordination with state, regional, and local plans and programs; that federal agencies be furnished with information on the relationship of proposed direct federal development projects and activities to state, regional, and local plans and programs, in order to assure maximum feasible consistency of federal developments with such plans and programs; and that federal agencies be provided with information concerning the possible impact of proposed federal developments on the environment.

Relationship Information Concerning State Plans: The next provision of OMB *Circular No. A-95* requires that federal agencies be furnished with information on the relationship of each state plan required under various federal programs to state comprehensive health plans and to other state plans.

Coordination of Planning in Multijurisdictional Areas: Finally, OMB *Circular No. A-95* establishes guidelines for the coordination of planning in multijurisdictional areas. It encourages and facilitates state and local initiative and responsibility for the development of organizational and procedural arrangements to coordinate comprehensive and functional activities; it calls for the elimination of overlap, duplication, and competition in those state and local planning activities that are federally assisted; it encourages the most effective use of state and local resources available for development planning; it calls for minimizing inconsistencies that exist among federal agencies and the approval requirements placed upon state, regional, and metropolitan development planning activities; and it encourages the states to exercise leadership in delineating and establishing a system of planning and to develop districts or regions in each state which can provide a consistent geographic base for the coordination of federal, state, and local development programs. This last point—that is, the geographic area covered by a program—is important because, prior to the designation of a planning district under any federal program, the federal agency procedures will provide for a review of its boundaries and will comment upon its relationship to planning districts already established by the state. These must conform unless there is clear justification for not doing so.

In many metropolitan areas, the designated clearinghouse is the Council of Governments (COG). In fact, the review process established under OMB

Circular No. A-95 is probably the only authority that the COGs can cite in their claim of regional governance responsibilities.

One of the problems with the A-95 review process has been that it is very difficult to fit locally proposed actions into regional plans since very few, if any, appropriate regional plans exist. This accounts for the usual review and comment conclusion, "This proposal is not inconsistent with regional planning." Another practical problem with the A-95 review process is that it usually takes several months to complete, which can be a delaying factor in the application cycle for grant awards.

The A-95 process, however, does have the potential to inform affected agencies in a region about a proposed action, and it is able to ensure a process of discussion that should result in maximization of the objectives of various concerned agencies. The clearinghouse function can become a major aspect of the federal system and can help to resolve many of the problems of the categorical grant programs. Another benefit of the A-95 process is that it requires the regional clearinghouse to notify all affected parties, including the local government, of the proposed action.

There seems to be a breakdown or, perhaps, a lack of interest in the whole process, since frequently there is no feedback from the federal level to the regional clearinghouses regarding actions resulting from comments upon applications.

Unfortunately, not all federal assistance programs fall under the requirements of OMB *Circular No. A-95*. Those that are covered, however, include specific programs of the Departments of Agriculture, Commerce, Defense, HEW, HUD, Interior, Justice, Labor, and Transportation; also, some programs of OEO, the National Science Foundation, the Water Resources Council, and the Appalachian Regional Commission. *Circular No. A-95* does not, by any means, cover all the programs of any of these agencies.[25,26]

[25] Mogulof, Melvin B. "Regional Planning, Clearance and Evaluation; A Look at the A–95 Process." *American Institute of Planners Journal*, 37(6):418–421, November 1971.
[26] Office of Management and Budget, Executive Office of the President. *Circular No. A–95* (Revised). Washington, D.C., U.S. Government Printing Office, 1971.

REFERENCES

1. American Hospital Association. *Statement on Planning for Hospital Construction in Small Communities.* Chicago, 1968. (No. 548)

2. Anderson, Donna and Anderson, Nancy N. *Comprehensive Health Planning in the States: A Current Status Report.* Minneapolis, Health Services Research Center, American Rehabilitation Foundation, 1969.

3. Arnold, Mary F. and Hink, Douglas L. "Agency Problems in Planning for Community Health Needs." *Medical Care,* 6:454–466, November–December 1968.

4. Brickman, Harry R. "Federal Versus Local Community Mental Health Planning: A Plea for Conflict Resolution." *American Journal of Public Health,* 60(12):2251–2256, December 1970.

5. Community Health, Inc. *The Voluntary Role in the Partnership for Health.* New York, 1969.

6. Conant, Ralph W. *The Politics of Community Health.* Report of the Community Action Studies Project, National Commission on Community Health Services. Washington, D.C., Public Affairs Press, 1968.

7. Curran, William J. "Health Planning Agencies: A Legal Crisis?" *American Journal of Public Health,* 60(2):359–360, February 1970.

8. Mott, B.J.F. *Anatomy of a Coordinating Council: Implications for Planning.* Pittsburgh, University of Pittsburgh Press, 1968.

9. P.L. 90–174. *Partnership for Health Amendments of 1967.* Washington, D.C., U.S. Government Printing Office, 1967.

10. P.L. 91–515. *Heart Disease, Cancer, Stroke, and Kidney Disease Amendments of 1970.* Washington, D.C., U.S. Government Printing Office, 1970.

11. Sigmond, Robert M. "Process or Outcome Planning—Which Concept Will Dominate?" *Hospital Topics,* June 1969, pp. 35–39.

12. Somers, Anne R. "Goals Into Reality: The Challenges of Health Planning." *Hospitals,* 43(Parts I and II):41–49, August 1, 1969.

13. Somers, Herman and Somers, Anne. *Medicare and the Hospitals.* Washington, D.C., The Brookings Institution, 1967. pp. 204–225.

14. Stebbins, Ernest L. and Williams, Kathleen N. "History and Background of Health Planning in the United States." In: Reinke, W.A. *Health Planning: Qualitative Aspects and Quantitative Techniques.* Baltimore, Waverly Press, Inc., 1972. pp. 10–13.

15. Stone, Lana B. *From Organization to Operation: The Evolving Areawide*

Comprehensive Health Planning Scene. Minneapolis, Health Services Research Center, American Rehabilitation Foundation, 1969.

16. U.S. Department of Health, Education, and Welfare, Health Services and Mental Health Administration, Office of Grants Management. *Profiles of Grant Programs*. 1971 Edition. Washington, D.C., U.S. Government Printing Office, 1971. (Stock Number 1720–0033)

17. U.S. Department of Housing and Urban Development. *Community Development Evaluation Series No. 3, Local Strategies to Affect State Plan Allocation of Federal Funds*. Washington, D.C., U.S. Government Printing Office, 1972.

CHAPTER 3

ORGANIZING FOR PLANNING

To say that planners and others involved in planning procedures seldom project a course of action for their own planning activities may appear to be an absurd statement, but in reality this is often true. The fact is that, unless planning is handled the same as any other purposeful enterprise, the results may be unsatisfactory. The purpose of this chapter, therefore, is to delineate some of the guidelines for the planning activity per se, to determine who should participate in a planning action, and to suggest how these participants should be selected.

DESCRIBING THE PLAN

A little reflection will quickly show that no two plans are the same; they come in all shapes, sizes, and varieties. Thus, it is necessary to define the nature of the planning effort under consideration. The definition then becomes the basis for deciding how planning will be done and who should participate in it.

Le Breton and Henning in their book, *Planning Theory*,[1] state that a plan has 13 dimensions. Specifically, these are: complexity, significance, comprehensiveness, time, specificity, completeness, flexibility, frequency, confidential nature, formality, authorization, ease of implementation, and ease of control. Each of these dimensions is further defined in their book, and there is some discussion concerning the implications of the presence or absence of each. Usually, it is not only a case of presence or absence of these dimensions, but also a matter of degree. For example, a plan may range from simple to highly complex, but it can seldom be classified at either extreme.

[1] Le Breton, Preston P. and Henning, Dale A. *Planning Theory*. Englewood Cliffs, N.J., Prentice-Hall, 1961. pp. 22–58, 160–244, 338–343.

Examples of the implications of these various dimensions in their relationship to a plan are listed below.

Dimensions	Implications
Complexity	Need for precise planning tools. More difficult coordination of planning activity.
Significance	Approval of plan moved to a higher level of authority. More people involved in planning.
Comprehensiveness	More people involved in planning. Greater problems in implementation of plans. Greater problems of control. More difficult coordination.
Time	Greater opportunity to pretest plan. Greater likelihood of changes in plan before it is implemented.
Specificity	Easier communication. Easier implementation. Easier coordination and control.
Completeness	Easier implementation. Greater chances of success.
Flexibility	Greater need for coordination.
Frequency	Greater likelihood of establishing a routine for the planning process.
Confidentiality	Minimum number of people involved in preparation and implementation of plans. Greater problems in collecting data for precise planning.
Formality	Easier acceptance by participants. Probable loss of flexibility with too much formality.
Authorization (Official Sanction)	Easier to obtain cooperation of participants. Entire planning process expedited.
Ease of Implementation	Shorter planning period.
Ease of Control	Responsibility for control placed at lower echelon within the organization.

These examples clearly indicate that quite often there will be countervailing forces. When this occurs, the person organizing the planning effort must make a subjective evaluation of•the relative importance of each dimension and weigh his decision accordingly.

Another approach to the planning process is that taken by Dror in his book, *Ventures in Policy Science*,[2] in which he lists five primary facets of planning. Each primary facet is subdivided into secondary facets, each secondary facet can be further subdivided into tertiary facets, and so on. Dror's primary facets of planning, and his examples of secondary facets, are as follows:

Primary	*Secondary*
A. General environment of the planning process.	Basic factors, for example, demography.
B. Resources available for planning and execution of the plan.	Limitations on planning, for example, power groups. Values. Terms of reference for planning, for example, general goals.
C. Subject matter of the planning process.	Relations between subject and planning unit. Elasticity of the subject matter. Degree of penetration. Significance of subject matter. Orientation of the subject for planning. Extent of previous planning and subject area. Scope of the activity planned. Territorial area that is planned. Time span to be allowed.
D. Planning unit itself.	Basic nature of the planning unit. Primary or dedicated planning units. Status of the planning unit. Values, information, character of the planning unit. Resources and needs of the planning unit. Work methods and procedures used in planning. Organizational structure of the planning unit.
E. Form of the plan to be arrived at.	Degree of realism required. Form of the plan, for example, time period work plan or contingency plan. Degree of detail for the plan.

2 Dror, Yehezkel. *Ventures in Policy Science*. New York, American Elsevier, 1971. pp. 108–116.

Clearly, these categories are too broad to be more than illustrative. Each one must be thought through for specific application to an individual plan. Furthermore, from Dror's listing, it can be inferred that the planning unit is taken as it is presented, whereas in the Le Breton and Henning approach, most of the items under Dror's category C will be the basis for the development of other categories.

In short, we are striving here for the application of a situational theory of planning. This implies that a single approach or theory is not appropriate for all situations. The planner must diagnose the situation in which he finds himself and then should use the approach that is most likely to succeed under the given circumstances.

ORGANIZATION FOR PLANNING

A review of broad-scale planning in the United States, discussed in more detail in Chapter 2, is not particularly encouraging. We find, for instance, that, at the national level, there is no such thing as a general health planning agency; rather, there are fragmented, programmatic organizations. For example, the Comprehensive Health Planning Service has little formal influence over the Hill-Burton program.

At the next lower level—the federal region—we find that a similar situation exists. A step forward has been the establishment of coincident boundaries among all federal programs, which has eliminated the overlapping that would occur when the federal regions of HEW were defined differently than the federal regions of other departments, such as HUD. The rationale for decentralization to these regional offices allows for greater input from the local level and concurrently offers greater understanding of the unique problems endemic to the various parts of the United States.

Offsetting these advantages are the problems encountered in a dilution of expertise: first, the number of federal specialists must be spread over a greater number of regional offices than would be necessary if decision making were concentrated at the national level. There is also some question of authority at the regional offices: Has decision making really been delegated to the regional level? Finally, there is the problem of ensuring consistency among the regions in the administration of national programs. As an example, consider the matter of consistency as an administrative problem:

Why should the review process for grants be more rigorous in one region than in another? Why should not all agencies receive the same treatment regardless of geographic location?

The lack of general coordinated planning also is found at the state level. State Comprehensive Health Planning (CHP) agencies were established under Section 314(a) (P.L. 89–749) to correct much of this difficulty; however, there are many reasons why this has not happened. For instance, quite often the CHP agency has been placed within the state health department; but, frequently, the jurisdiction of health departments does not include all of the health activities within the state. Furthermore, being within the health department often makes it difficult to coordinate with nonhealth activities that are vital to comprehensive health programs. Some states have exercised their option to place the CHP agency in the governor's office. This can solve some of the problems of fragmentation, but it also raises other issues that relate to maintaining a sense of community interest with the state agencies that have primary responsibility for delivery of health services.

Moving from the state level to the local or areawide level, things become even more chaotic. Here, in addition to the problem of vertical fragmentation of programs and departments, we find that there is a great deal of what might be called horizontal fragmentation, due to the multiplicity of local jurisdictions. One might call this the "1,400 governments syndrome," which is the name of a study of the New York metropolitan region that counted 1,400 political jurisdictions within that one area.[3] The planning agency that attempts to bring all these jurisdictions together at the local level is the 314(b) agency—commonly called the areawide Comprehensive Health Planning agency. Clearly, this agency faces an uphill battle all the way. It generally has no formal authority over the activities of the various political jurisdictions within its area, and it has no direct authority over the activities of the individual health providers that function within the region for which the CHP (314(b)) agency is responsible.

Another problem, especially at the local level, is the unwillingness of people to consider the entire spectrum of health problems. There is a strong tendency for planning agencies to focus on personal health services to the exclusion of environmental health problems and, even more often, to focus on health facility planning because of familiarity with this particular aspect of planning. A notable effort to overcome some of these difficulties is evident in

[3] Wood, Robert C. *1400 Governments Syndrome.* Cambridge, Mass., Harvard University Press, 1961.

those areas where the areawide health planning agency is a part of a regional agency, such as a metropolitan council of governments or a regional planning council, which concerns itself with all planning activities within the area.

INTERNAL PLANNING ORGANIZATION

Having taken a brief overview of the broad organization for planning, from federal through state and, finally, through local levels, the next step to be considered is the organization of a specific planning unit. This unit may be within a health institution, such as a hospital, or it may be a health planning agency per se.

One of the primary considerations is the manner in which the chief decision maker within the organization operates, specifically, his opinion of where planning should be done. At one end of the spectrum, the chief decision maker regards planning as something that he, personally, must do. At the opposite end of the spectrum, there is an institutionalized planning unit that receives only general guidance from the chief executive.

It is important to note that, under a tightly controlled planning process, it is likely that innovation will occur only when outside pressures are placed upon the executive. When more than one person is involved in the planning process, however, the average rate of innovation will be higher, and that rate will tend to be constant. It should be noted also that, regardless of which planning style is adopted, responsibility for the planning function must remain at the top level of the organization. It is less delegable than other management functions because of the great danger of suboptimization in the use of scarce resources. Therefore, regardless of how much the chief decision maker may want to delegate the planning function, it remains his responsibility to ensure that all plans are coordinated and integrated into a rational total plan.

OPTIONS FOR A PLANNING UNIT

Various options for a planning unit are available to the chief decision maker if he decides that someone other than himself should carry out the planning functions. We will consider, here, four separate options for implementing the planning function.

Governing Board and Committees of the Board: If the organization's governing body is to perform the planning function, then the plans can deal only with the most complex, comprehensive, and significant problems. This type of planning is usually done in very broad terms unless subcommittees are formed and an adequate staff is provided. The latter procedure is very common in health planning agencies, and it frequently appears in health institutions as well. One of the major advantages in using the subcommittee arrangement is that it provides an excellent way to get the advice and consent of the external-interest groups who are invited to participate in the planning process. This benefit can be increased by expanding the membership of subcommittees to include persons who are not members of the governing board of the organization. Thus, one can have a multitude of committees, each having a minimum of one member from the formal governing board of the organization, with the remainder of the membership being comprised of representatives of affected groups and/or professional experts.

Committees of Chief Operating Officials: This option applies mostly within an institution. It could, however, occur in a health planning agency if the committees are comprised of providers of particular types of services, such as a committee of nursing home administrators.

If a committee of this scope itself does the planning, the plans will tend to be broad and not very specific. These generally are very busy individuals, and they have neither the time nor the inclination to concern themselves with the minute details necessary for the final implementation of a plan. If, however, the members of this committee are not of the decision-making echelon, but rather are subordinates, then the committee may lack authority to make the commitments necessary to carry out the plan.

The primary advantage of this particular style of planning—that is, where the chief operating officials act as the decision makers—is that it allows the persons who will be directly affected by the plan, and who probably have the greatest amount of expertise in the functions involved, to participate in the planning. Furthermore, their participation increases the likelihood that they will accept the plans which eventually evolve.

One way to offset the tendency of such a committee to avoid detail is to organize a committee of key decision makers and then provide it with a project organization that will do all the specific detailed planning that is necessary—subject, of course, to the approval of the committee itself.

Planning by Committee: Another choice is to have the planning function executed by a planning committee with membership other than governing boards or operating officials. Since the committee plays such a vital role in the planning process, let us examine some of the considerations involved in the establishment of a committee.

Committees may be of several types. *A control committee* in effect acts as a pluralistic decision maker. An *advisory committee* merely evaluates the proposals of others. Finally, an *investigative and advisory committee* initiates actions and develops recommendations for solutions; note, however, that it does not have the authority to implement those recommendations.

To be effective, a committee must have authority commensurate with its role. It must be staffed with good members and supported by adequate technical assistance. Finally, it must have a clear charter, or it will spend all of its time deciding what it is supposed to do.

The committee approach to planning has a number of important advantages. The first of these is the ability to achieve informal but effective coordination among members representing the diverse interests affected by the plan. Second, this diversity of membership brings a wider range of knowledge to apply to the problem at hand. As noted earlier, participants tend to accept solutions by groups of which they are members. Finally, and significantly, a skilled executive can use the committee as a delaying device when it is necessary to prevent someone or some group from initiating an ill-conceived or premature project.

This same delaying process, of course, represents one of the most significant disadvantages of committee activity. Committees tend to be very slow and quite expensive, while time is of the essence in the planning process. For example, given the problems of inflation, postponement of decisions frequently involves a substantial increase in the cost of a project. Another disadvantage is that committees tend to develop compromise decisions. Consensus is not necessarily optimum. Finally, responsibility for the activities of the committee cannot effectively be placed on any one individual. Even the chairman of the committee can easily rationalize delaying tactics and indecisiveness by attributing the problems to other members of the group.

Staff Planning Groups: The final option that will be considered here is the staff planning group, which is an alternative to the committee approach when an executive wishes to delegate some of the work involved in the planning process. The advantages and disadvantages are essentially the reverse of those described for planning by committees. The biggest drawback to planning by staff groups is the potential for noninvolvement of those people who will be most directly affected by the plan. The greatest advantage is that a specific person is assigned the primary responsibility for implementing the planning process. Such a person may be regarded as an integrator of organizational functions.[4] This requires a staff of especially talented people, who are very expensive and hard to find. The integrator must be a person who contributes to decisions on the basis of his expertise rather than his position. He must have a balanced orientation between operation and development, between service and cost, and between specialty concerns and the total plan. He also must be acceptable as an arbitrator of interorganizational disputes, which will inevitably arise in the planning process. Ignoring these disputes, hiding conflicts, or using arbitrary measures simply will not work. Each of these tactics tends to be successful on an immediate basis, but eventually will destroy the effectiveness of the planning process.

Once the chief decision maker has determined who will perform the work involved in the planning process, then that planning group must decide which type of planning organization will be set up—the project organization or the task force.

PROJECT ORGANIZATION[5]

The project organization (or project unit) can be used alone or to support a committee. It should be used when there is an important task that requires special attention for an extended period of time and which involves an interdepartmental or interagency effort. There are four kinds of project organizations:

1. *Individual project unit*, in which one person exercises control through operating units that are performing the work.
2. *Staff project unit*, wherein a project manager has a staff that exercises control over operating units through budgets, schedules, etc., but requires that all of the actual planning be done by the operating units.
3. *Intermix project units*, in which some functions are performed by the

---

4 Lawrence, Paul R. and Lorsch, Jay W. "New Management Job: The Integrator." *Harvard Business Review*, 45(6):142–151, November–December 1967.
5 Middleton, C.J. "How to Set Up a Project Organization." *Harvard Business Review*, 45(2):73–82, March–April 1967.

operating units previously described, and some are performed by the project staff.

4. *Aggregate project unit*, in which the project manager has direct control of all the activities required to complete the project, whether these activities are assigned to the planning group or to the operating units.

The project unit offers several advantages: it gives better control over and provides for faster accomplishment of the project; it tends to lower project costs; it brings more skills to apply to the problem at hand; and, because of participation by those involved, it tends to make the outcome more acceptable.

The project unit also presents some disadvantages: primarily it does not develop a pool of expertise that can be drawn upon when similar tasks arise in the future; also, it tends to disrupt the other operations of the organization. In effect, it results in splitting the responsibility between the project manager—who has little concern with the day-to-day operation—and the functional manager—who has slight interest in the achievement of the particular project. For the same reason, functional managers tend to withhold their best resources—especially people—from participation in the project; those people who do participate suffer the anxieties inherent in having two supervisors with different interests.

TASK FORCE

The task force is a variant of the project organization. Typically, its time span tends to be shorter than that of a project organization. It is usually formed by borrowing people from operating units. When this is done, jobs should be held open within the operating units for those people who have been assigned temporarily to the task force so that their jobs will not be in jeopardy. This type of planning organization tends to be less disruptive than the project organization, since the people participating in the task force are removed from the day-to-day operation of the organization.

There are several advantages to the task force approach. First, it provides a wider range of expertise than can be obtained with a full-time planning staff. Second, it offers opportunities for representation and participation. Of particular importance is the fact that it facilitates coordination of all the subplans as they affect the various departments, because the representatives of these subplans are members of the task force. Also, the departmental or agency representatives receive training in planning, and they take this knowledge (both of planning in general and of the specific plan which is developed) back to their regular jobs in the operating units, thereby providing an infusion of expertise to their parent units. Finally, the task force provides for optimum utilization of scarce personnel resources because of the varying level of the workload in planning for any specific function. (See Figure 1.)

Figure 1 shows how planning for a particular project begins at a very low level and reaches a peak at implementation; it then gradually tapers off into a maintenance function, thus ensuring that the project will continue until such time as another innovation occurs, when a repetition of the cycle will begin. For example, a hospital probably does not need continuous planning for emergency services, but the emergency services offered must be periodically reassessed and improved upon. On the other hand, the planning staff must be kept fully occupied. This can be achieved by scheduling the planning of

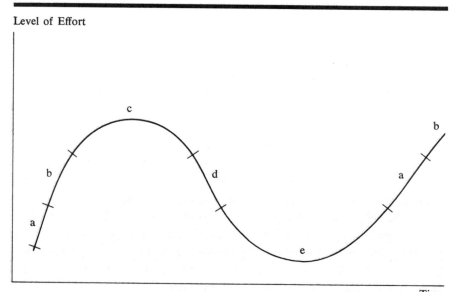

a—Initiation of New System
b—System Development
c—System Implementation
d—System Evaluation and Modification
e—System Maintenance

Figure 1:   Life cycle of a system

Level of Effort

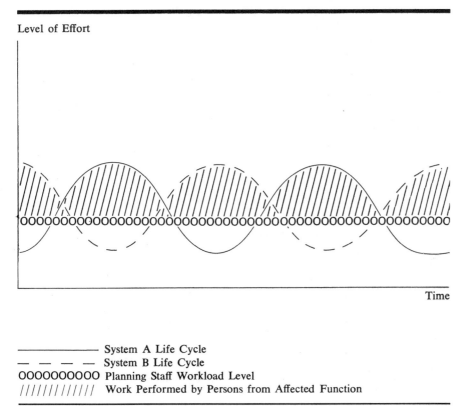

Time

—————————— System A Life Cycle
— — — — System B Life Cycle
OOOOOOOOOO Planning Staff Workload Level
///////////// Work Performed by Persons from Affected Function

Figure 2:   Maintenance of level of workload by phasing systems' life cycles

several projects so that as one diminishes to the maintenance stage, another is approaching the peak of activity in the implementation stage. The resulting workload of the planning staff is constant, and peak demands in planning for any function may be met by drawing personnel temporarily from the function being planned. Figure 2 is a simple two-plan diagram showing how this could be accomplished. Obviously, in the real world there are many more types of plans to coordinate, but the general concept is illustrated in this diagram.

ORGANIZATIONAL SUMMARY

Up to this point, we have demonstrated that planning can be performed in a variety of modes, depending upon the style of the chief decision maker. It is fairly safe to say that little planning will be performed when the chief decision maker himself takes the sole responsibility for this particular function. It is virtually inevitable that pressing, day-to-day activities will take priority over those that are seen as postponable; consequently, planning will be generally neglected. Thus, when no one person has the primary responsibility for planning per se, then this function tends to be postponed to a point where it is no longer planning, but rather becomes a frantic reaction to an incipient crisis. If a decision maker accepts this analysis, his problem then becomes one of determining how to organize so that effective planning will be conducted on a consistent and continuous basis. There are several alternative organizational arrangements that he might consider. The first of these is the committee approach, for which he may use the governing board, committees of the board, operating officials, or any other group that he feels is competent. If the committee approach has too many disadvantages for the type of planning he has decided to undertake, he may consider the establishment of a separate planning group, which could be a staff or a line organization. Again he has a choice between alternatives—the project organization or the task force.

This concludes the discussion of the organizational pattern by which the chief decision maker may set up a planning procedure based on his own internal resources. The following is a discussion of supplementary resources, that is, the use of outside consultants where special expertise is called for.

SUPPLEMENTARY RESOURCES

To implement the planning function, the chief executive may also consider the possibility of augmenting his own internal resources by using an outside consultant. Consultants in the planning field basically are people who have special knowledge which they can contribute to the planning process. This special knowledge usually is derived from a very high level of education and intensive experience within a very limited scope of activities.

The use of consultants is a fairly common practice within the health industry. This can be attributed to a number of things. First, health agencies, historically, have lacked expertise in managerial and administrative functions. Even in a well-staffed organization, consultants can be used to provide skills which simply are not available within the organization because such skills are not required on a continuing basis in its day-to-day operations. Second, very few health agencies have adequate staffing to perform more than their day-to-day operational functions. The consultant is another source of manpower that the chief decision maker may use when a planning project unit or task force would divert too many man-days from ongoing operations.

Consultants may do anything from creating the entire plan to carrying out a very specific assignment related to one small segment of the plan. For example, a general consultant might produce an entire plan, whereas an architect would convert the functional plan into a construction plan and supervise its implementation.

Some of the most common functions of consultants are: identifying the need for a plan, that is, establishing organizational objectives; gathering data for a plan and then analyzing the data; developing alternatives and evaluating these alternatives; or simply evaluating plans which have been developed by others. In summary, the foregoing list is essentially a recapitulation of the planning process. A consultant may accomplish any or all of these steps.

We must not, however, overlook some very important contributions that consultants can make, including their capability to sell a plan. It is widely acknowledged that no man can be a prophet in his own country; therefore, it is often necessary to have outside, "unbiased" experts as the authors of proposals before such propositions will be accepted by the persons who will be affected. Then, too, implementation of a plan often requires special knowledge and experience which may not be available within an organization because the specific function may not occur frequently. A good example is supervision of construction. Architects do this with great skill because they have had experience on similar projects. An individual hospital has construction projects under way only at very infrequent intervals, therefore, is at a disadvantage in this area.

SELECTION OF CONSULTANTS

The use of consultants creates very special problems for the chief decision maker, all of which revolve around the selection of persons who are competent, ethical, and not inclined toward self-interest. A limited amount of free consultation may be obtained by dealing with manufacturers' representatives. Needless to say, these agents do not meet the criterion of disinterestedness, since they have something to sell; but they are competent and, for the most part, ethical. So the decision maker can get a certain amount of free input to the planning process if he carefully observes the dictum of *caveat emptor*.

Once the decision maker determines that he may have to go beyond the free contributions of manufacturers' representatives, he must then consider explicitly the conditions existing within his institution that necessitate engaging outside consultants. The following list[6] suggests the most important of these conditions:

1. Available staff lacks well-rounded experience.
2. Needed specialists are not available internally.
3. Additional staff and training time are not available.
4. Project involves a total organization survey.
5. Project is a broad study going beyond the organization.
6. Project requires advanced special techniques.
7. Outside appraisal, "sales" assistance, or experience from other businesses is desired.

To save time, the decision maker should make his selection of a consultant in a phased mode or a series of steps. These probably would include a preliminary investigation, followed by an RFP (Request for Proposal) and an evaluation of the RFP responses, including a reference check of the consultants.

THE PRELIMINARY INVESTIGATION

At the outset, the decision maker should define—in clear and precise terms —the exact nature of the project he wishes to undertake. This will determine, to a large extent, the kinds of firms he should contact. He should then identify a number of persons or firms he feels would be interested and qualified to participate in the proposed project and should conduct rather informal but, nevertheless, specific interviews with each of these firms. There are many kinds of consulting firms; some have highly specialized staffs and function only in very limited areas, whereas others have broad skills and can offer a wide range of consulting talents.

Good sources of information for this preliminary investigation would be professional associations and other health agencies that have conducted simi-

[6] Haslett, J.W. "Decision Table for Engaging a Consultant." *Journal of Systems Management,* 22(7):12–14, July 1971.

lar projects in the recent past. Once the initial list of contenders is compiled, the decision maker should determine the following points for each:

1. The history of the company.
2. The background of its personnel.
3. Its financial status.
4. Its cooperativeness, or how easy it has been to work with in the past.
5. Its inventiveness. (Does it come up with new ideas, or is there a distinct impression that it has predetermined solutions for problems that might develop?)
6. The number and type of satisfied clients, and the amount of repeat business the company receives from its former clients.
7. The pertinence of the consulting company's specific experience to the project that the decision maker has in mind (most consultants have broad expertise and, in terms of knowledge, may legitimately claim to have relevant skills; however, in terms of the kind of experience the decision maker is looking for, this may not be the case).
8. Each consulting firm under consideration should be required to give some preliminary information about its fee arrangements. Are operations based on a fixed price, a time-and-materials cost basis, a retainer fee, or some other kind of arrangement?

Any consulting company that fails to meet these preliminary screening criteria should be immediately eliminated. Firms that just manage to meet these criteria also should be excluded from further consideration.

REQUEST FOR PROPOSAL

Once the field of contenders has been determined, the qualified firms should be invited to discuss the project in more detail. The project specifications should be given to all contenders to enable each to submit a formal proposal for the service to be performed. These specifications should be submitted in a formal document so there will be no ambiguity about what is expected. This is often called an RFP (Request for Proposal). The RFP should clearly identify the nature of the problem and the objectives of the project. It also should state the mandatory requirements and desired capabilities that will be the criteria for judging the qualifications of the competing companies and their proposed approaches to the problems. Stated more explicitly, the RFP must require that each bidder cover the following points in his proposal:

1. A restatement of his understanding of specific project objectives.
2. His technical approach.
3. The staff that will be allocated to the project (this is particularly important because very often consultants have been hired on the basis of the principal's qualifications; then later it has been discovered that the principal seldom, if ever, contributed to the study of the problem).
4. A specific time schedule.
5. Cost factors, including the method of billing.
6. The consulting firm's methods of project control and status reporting.
7. Specific areas of responsibilities that the consultant will assume, as well as those areas of the project for which he disclaims all responsibility.
8. The assistance that the consultant will require from the hiring agency.
9. The contractual terms and conditions under which the proposal is offered.
10. References from satisfied clients.

EVALUATION OF RFP RESPONSES

The third step in the selection of a consultant is an evaluation of the responses to the RFP, including reference checking. Three areas are of special importance to the decision maker: adequacy of the technical features of the proposal, the fee asked by the consulting organization, and the qualifications of the consultant.

The first step in the evaluation process is to determine the performance history of the consultants, particularly among agencies having backgrounds on similar projects. This is a difficult undertaking because, obviously, agencies are reluctant to admit having made serious errors. Consequently, the reference checker must be prepared to do some probing by asking questions such as the following: What kind of work did the firm do? Was it done completely and on time? Were the solutions practical and economical? Did the assigned personnel perform competently and objectively? How did the assigned personnel work with the client staff? Did the firm's supervisory personnel spend adequate time controlling and supervising the project? Would the reference hire the same consulting firm for similar work or for a different kind of technical endeavor?

At this point, it must be stressed that the decision maker should not be reluctant to shop around. Consultant services will represent a substantial investment; therefore, he must get as much as possible for the limited dollars he will have to spend. This can be accomplished most advantageously by a careful analysis of the capabilities of each person or firm competing for the contract.

In fairness to the consultants, however, it must be pointed out, first, that the fundamental issue in determining the success or failure of a consulting project is how well the client agency has specified its goals and objectives. Without these, the consulting firm will achieve the desired objectives only by accident or with luck, or by investing a major portion of its time in trying to determine what the client's objectives are. Second, the client will be unable to evaluate the proposals unless he knows exactly what kind of services he is seeking. Because of the nature of the consultant's relationship to the health agency, it is often desirable to go beyond the formal written proposals and engage in a selection process involving face-to-face presentation of proposals by the competing consultants. The evaluation of these proposals then is made by the chief decision maker with the advice and guidance of his staff or board of directors.

USE OF CONSULTANTS

The chief decision maker's responsibility does not end with the selection of the consultant. Realizing that a consultant's time is a very valuable and costly resource, he must do everything within his power to ensure that it is used most economically, particularly: by providing facilities for the consultant's personnel while they are working on the premises of the client organization; by making arrangements to meet with persons in affected groups; and by introducing his own staff and facilitating their contact with the staff of the consulting agency. There should be no indecision or reluctance on the part of the client's staff to assist the consultant in complete accordance with the terms of the contract.

Finally, the chief decision maker must carefully examine the periodic reports submitted by the consultant, thereby ensuring that reasonable progress is being made and that the progress is in the desired direction. It is easy to imagine the recriminations that can occur when, after the consultant has submitted monthly status reports that have been accepted without comment for a period of a year, the client voices dissatisfaction with the approach to the problem, or with the results accomplished. The consultant might be somewhat to blame for having accepted silence as indicative of approval, but, obviously, the major portion of the blame must be placed on the client.

REFERENCES

1. Branch, Melville. *Planning Aspects and Applications.* New York, Wiley, 1966. pp. 56–58.
2. Carner, Donald C. *Planning for Hospital Expansion.* Springfield, Ill., C.C. Thomas, 1968. pp. 23–26.
3. Hallahan, Fred. "If You Don't Know Who's In Charge, the Hospital Will Look Like It." *Modern Hospital, 114*(4):108–110, April 1970.
4. Hudenberg, Roy. *Planning the Community Hospital.* New York, McGraw-Hill, 1967. pp. 43–57.
5. Mason, R. Hal. "Developing a Planning Organization." *Business Horizons, 12*(4):61–69, August 1969.
6. McGibony, John R. *Principles of Hospital Administration.* 2nd Edition. New York, Putnam, 1952. pp. 54–65.
7. Wrapp, H. Edward. "Organization for Long-Range Planning." *Harvard Business Review, 35* (1):27–47, January-February 1957.

CHAPTER 4

FORECASTING

THE FORECAST

Planning may be defined as making current decisions in the light of future expectations, which implies that the future may be different from the present. Therefore, in order to plan adequately, we must have some idea of how the future will look; we must forecast the environment in which we will be operating during the period for which we are planning.

To develop a forecast, two things are required: First, the planners must prepare a description of the specific situation for the projected planning period; this is the forecast content. Second, the planners must explain how the situation will evolve from its current state into the forecast state; this points up the advantages of forecast preparation. For example, if we were to predict that the proportion of aged persons in a community would increase dramatically over a period of 10 years, then we might go on to state that this would occur because of an economic decline within that community. Such a decline would drive out the young people who normally would be in the labor force, thus leaving the community with a residual of elderly persons. The net effect of this change would be that the absolute size of the population might decrease, but the proportion of elderly within that decreased population figure would be substantially larger.

FORECAST CONTENT

The forecast content must cover all aspects of situations in which we expect to be planning. It should be both qualitative and quantitative; it might contain the average expected conditions, or it might show a range of possible outcomes. Quite often, because of uncertainties, it will be necessary to provide the decision maker with several alternative outcomes. He will have to decide, on the basis of his subjective assessment of probabilities, which alternative is the most likely to occur, and then act accordingly.

As noted above, the forecast must contain projections for the planning

61

period, as well as a statement of current conditions. Furthermore, the forecast is not merely a catalog of facts; it must interpret the facts relating to current conditions in terms of their significance for the health of the community. In this respect, absolute and relative numbers are frequently inadequate descriptors; the planner must also consider spatial and temporal relationships. For example: Where are the health centers located in relation to the population? How has physician supply changed during the last 10 years?

If a forecast is to cover adequately the many factors affecting the health of a community, it should include six major components. Each component should reflect current status, basis for forecasting, and expected state at the end of the planning period. These components are outlined in Figure 3;

Specific Forecast Components

A. Political

    1. Jurisdictions*
    2. Governments
      a. Official Health Agencies

B. Social

    1. Population Size and Composition
      a. Age, Race, Sex
    2. Education
    3. Housing
    4. Ethnicity
    5. Mobility

C. Economic

    1. Major Sources of Employment
    2. Occupations and Income
    3. Natural Resources
    4. Transportation Systems
    5. Land Use

D. Technological

    1. Health Services Technology
    2. Environmental Management
      Technology

E. Health (Personal)

    1. Health Resources
      a. Facilities
      b. Manpower
        (1) Education and Training
      c. Funds
    2. Health Status
      a. Mortality
      b. Morbidity
    3. Health Services
      a. Existing Services
        (1) Availability
        (2) Utilization
        (3) Effect
        (4) Adequacy
        (5) Efficiency
      b. Needed Services

F. Health (Environmental)

    1. General Subject (e.g., water quality)
      a. Current Status and Impact
      b. Existing Programs
        (1) Criteria
        (2) Procedures
        (3) Resources
        (4) Constraints

* The general content for this and each specific component outlined should be: current status, trends and other bases for forecasting, and expected state.

Figure 3:   Outline of the forecast content

however, the items enumerated under each component are suggestive rather than comprehensive. A brief explanation of each component follows:

Political: should describe the health decision-making individuals, organizations, and processes; both official and unofficial elements should be included.
Social: should provide a description of the community population.
Economic: should include geographic and communications information as well as traditional economic factors.
Technological: should comprise forecasts of the state of technology that will prevail in health, environmental management, economic activities, and services during the planning period.
Personal Health: should cover health status of the population, health resources available, and health services—both existing and required.
Environmental Health: should contain a separate discussion of each major environmental component, but relationships between components should also be described.

FORECAST PREPARATION

In preparing a forecast, planners have an opportunity to discuss the future, with the concurrent advantage of developing a factual statement of expectations for the future. Such a statement will crystallize the assumptions being made, thus eliminating fuzzy or inconsistent expectations; will make these expectations or assumptions explicit, thus facilitating communications with others, as well as review by the decision maker; and will clarify the criteria which should be used in the evaluation. For example, infant mortality rate would be an inappropriate health-status indicator if genetic engineering were to be widely adopted.

Having reviewed the general content of the basic description, we will now consider the techniques—general and specific—available for making a forecast within each particular area of consideration.

GENERAL FORECASTING TECHNIQUES

There is no widespread agreement as to the exact number of known forecasting techniques. Daniel Bell[1] has identified 12; others say that there are as

---

[1] Bell, Daniel. "Twelve Modes of Predictions—A Preliminary Sorting of Approaches in the Social Science." *Daedalus, 93*(2):847–868, Spring 1964.

many as 100. The methods which Bell identifies appear to be adequate for our purposes. They are:

1. *Social Physics:* This technique is exemplified by such things as the learning curve and the concept of marginal utility.
2. *Trends and Forecasts:* These processes consist of straight-line, exponential, or cyclical extrapolations which generally do not seek to discover underlying causes.
3. *Structural Certainties:* These factors are based upon laws and customs. For example: In a presidential election, the party in power usually nominates the incumbent unless he is in his second term of office.
4. *Operational Code:* This mode of prediction is based upon the life-style or the character of a group. For example: Southern white people generally are expected to be conservative.
5. *Operational System:* This mechanism is an effort to specify the underlying sources of power in a society, regardless of momentary fluctuations of office holding. Understanding these power sources leads to the ability of determining how they will attempt to direct the movement of society. It should be emphasized that there may be many coexisting operational systems; for example, a property-based system, an education-based system, and a politically based system may function side by side.
6. *Structural Requisites:* These factors often are used to show the limits that might be anticipated. For example, gross national product cannot grow at more than 5 percent per year due to the limited supply of available manpower.
7. *Overriding Problem:* In this technique, the forecaster identifies an issue of such importance that all other actions are designed to deal with it. For example, we might say that poverty overrides; consequently, health programs, education programs, and housing programs concentrate on means of reducing poverty. In the health area, this would result in employment of indigenous personnel to provide health services.
8. *Prime Mover:* If one factor is identified as an independent variable, then other variables will follow it. For example, increasing racial integration will cause changes in many other activities, such as education and recreation.
9. *Sequential Development:* This forecasting technique deals with limitations imposed by necessary preconditions. For example, Y cannot occur until X is finished.

10. *Accounting Schemes:* These processes consist of categorization of important factors with regard to the type of change that these factors normally would undergo, such as linear, cyclical, or unpredictable.

11. *Alternative Futures:* This method requires the forecaster to imagine the possibilities open to man and, then, to create a fiction. This has been done both by popular writers—for example, George Orwell, *1984*—and scientific technicians—for example, Herman Kahn, *The Year 2000.*

12. *Decision-Theory:* This approach involves the use of a variety of relatively new techniques, such as linear programming, game theory, and simulation. Many of these techniques are not yet developed to the point where they are suitable for practical application; and those that have been developed to this extent, such as linear programming and simulation, must be used with caution, for the forecaster should not use them in the normative sense. His role is to forecast what might happen, and, quite frequently, these tools are used for normative purposes.

A more condensed list of five methods was prepared and illustrated by Martin V. Jones of The MITRE Corporation.[2] His list, which is self-explanatory because of the samples provided, is shown in Figure 4.

Regardless of which approach to forecasting is taken, it is evident that the planner still faces the crucial problem of obtaining accurate data on which to base his forecast. A review of the aforementioned forecasting techniques reveals that many of the inputs are the judgments of individuals who might be considered experts. Indeed, in the past, there have been some examples of grossly inadequate technical forecasts that were based on just such expert opinion. For example, one inventor of electronic computers once said that six of these devices would be able to handle all of the business needs of the United States, which clearly indicates that unguided judgment or intuition is not really satisfactory for forecasting. To surmount this difficulty, a number of analysts at The RAND Corporation have attempted to improve the quality of judgmental input by developing a systematic forecasting method known as the Delphi Technique. In our scheme, it would appear that this technique fits the category of general forecasting techniques and, thus, may be used with any of the specific components of forecasting that were outlined in Figure 3. It is more readily adaptable, however, and thus more often used, in the area of technological forecasting; therefore, we will treat it in that sense later in

[2] Jones, Martin V. *Technology Assessment Methodology: Some Basic Propositions.* Washington, D.C., The Mitre Corporation, 1971. 127 pp. MTR 6009, Vol. 1, PB 202 778–01.

FORECASTING METHODS

DEFINITION	EXAMPLE
INTUITION A forecast based on the subjective judgment of the forecaster.	Experts at an extemporaneous workshop session of a joint physician, computer-industry symposium predict that by 1985 approximately 65% of U. S. physicians will employ computer diagnostic services. They cite as evidence the increasing experimentation with the use of automated techniques in the medical profession.
TREND EXTRAPOLATION A forecast based on the assumption of the continuation into the future of some discerned past trend.	Statistics show that over the past 15 years the percentage of physicians using computer diagnostic services increased from 4 to 27%. Continuing that trend for the next 15 years indicates that by 1985 approximately 65% of physicians will employ computer diagnostic services.
TREND CORRELATION A forecast of the future status of some phenomenon in terms of a consistent relationship of that phenomenon to some other phenomenon in the past whose future status has already been projected.	Historical data covering the last 10 years show that the percentage of physicians with access to computer diagnostic consultation is well correlated with three other factors: the increase in private group medical practice, the percentage of the population covered by medical insurance, and the percentage of doctors graduated from medical schools offering instruction in medical applications of computers. Projections on these three factors are available through 1985. Using these projections as a basis, a statistical correlation analysis indicates that by 1985 65% of physicians will have access to computer diagnostic consultation.
MODELS (STATISTICAL) This method is a much elaborated version of the historical trend correlation technique described above. It often involves the use of dozens, and sometimes of hundreds, of estimating equations--all integrated into a unified forecasting method.	An in depth study of physicians who have already adopted computer diagnostic consultation services shows that such usage is related in a complex way to some 10 different variables such as physician work load, degree of medical specialization, the access to and use of other consultative services, the cost of the computer service, etc. Well documented studies make it possible to predict the growth factor through 1985 for these 10 governing variables. Using this later study and the cited historical relationship, it is possible to predict that 65% of physicians will employ computer diagnostic consultation in 1985.
ANALOGY This method predicts the future by drawing a plausible parallel between the future and some presumably similar prior event.	In terms of many management and scientific services the medical research field has been about 25 years ahead of the practicing physician. In 1960 approximately 65% of the nation's medical research facilities were using computers for data analysis and synthesis tasks similar to those involved in physician computer diagnostic consultation. On this basis it is predicted that by 1985 approximately 65% of physicians will employ computer diagnostic consultation services.

Reprinted by kind permission of The Mitre Corporation.

Figure 4: A recap of forecasting methods (Hypothetical question: What percentage of U.S. physicians will use computer diagnostic services by 1985?)

this chapter, following the discussion on Technological Forecasting. Although the Delphi Technique, in its original form, probably exceeds the resources and requirements of most health planners, it can nevertheless be adapted to meet the needs of almost any planning situation in any type of organization.

SPECIFIC FORECASTING TECHNIQUES

Although it is possible to envision how the previously described general techniques could be applied to any of the components in the forecast, it will be useful to examine a number of more specific approaches which have been developed to deal with the requirements for various types of forecasts. Four specific forecasting techniques are reviewed here in considerable detail.

POLITICAL FORECASTING

Current political forecasting is almost entirely lacking in formal forecasting processes; virtually all forecasts are now made on the basis of intuition and judgment. These can best be improved through application of some variation of the Delphi Technique. For example, Dror suggested a process for estimating political feasibility. His methodology employs the Delphi Technique using politicians, business executives, and citizens who are thought to be politically astute. Dror also suggests a methodology for forecasting the domestic political situation, which includes the use of a number of matrices; however, at the present time, there are no reported cases in which Dror's matrices have been applied.[3]

ECONOMIC FORECASTING

Economic projection methods have been thoroughly described in both professional and popular publications; therefore, only a quick overview of the five most common approaches will be given here.

1. The first category of economic projection might be called the *naive model*. This can take one of several forms. The most simplistic approach is to assume no change, which is implicit when planning without making a forecast. Nevertheless, it could also be the result achieved after careful analysis of the environment. Another rather naive model is one that as-

3 Dror, Yehezkel. *Ventures in Policy Sciences.* New York, American Elsevier, 1971. pp. 69–92.

sumes a proportional change, that is, everything increases by X percent per annum.

2. The second method is known as *time series analysis* and is a somewhat more sophisticated economic approach to forecasting. The analysis of a time series of data would indicate trends, cyclical variations, seasonal variations, and residual irregular events. Two of the specific techniques which can be employed are moving averages and least squares.

3. A third method of economic projection is the *barometric technique,* which is based upon the use of data that seem to be associated with the phenomenon in which we are interested. Thus, we find that there are leading indicators or events which tend to precede changes in the area of interest, and, in addition, there also can be coincident or lagging indicators.

4. The *opinion poll* is a fourth method of economic projection, an example of which is the McGraw-Hill capital spending projection, based upon an opinion poll of industrial leaders throughout the country.

5. The fifth category of economic projection techniques is the *mathematical model,* which can be rather simple, single equation models; more complex, simultaneous equation models; or even dynamic models that permit a study of the effect of each period of activity upon the next following period. A most useful, but rather rare, economic projection device is the input/output model, which divides the economy of the region into production and consumption sectors. By varying the coefficients in this table, it is possible to see how a change in one sector may have marked effects on other sectors throughout the region.

Since these mathematical models generally are costly and difficult to develop, very few health planners will have an opportunity to use them. Therefore, only when some other agency has developed such models for its own purpose can health planners expect to have these kinds of data available to them. An opportunity of this nature could occur when a health planning area has boundaries which are coincident with a regional body, such as an economic development district; however, for the most part, the health planner will have to make economic forecasts on the basis of less sophisticated techniques.

SOCIAL FORECASTING—POPULATION PROJECTION
Social forecasting is a combination of qualitative and quantitative approaches. The qualitative approaches deal with such things as attitudes,

values, and social systems. The quantitative data are found primarily in the areas of population and housing—the same data which ordinarily are covered by the Census. Unfortunately, the Census is taken only at 10-year intervals; therefore, the planner generally is forced to make an adjustment to census data in order to determine the current status and then to make a projection from that adjusted data for the period for which he is planning. In this section, we will concentrate on projections of population—that is, the quantitative approach, since it usually is the key independent variable in health planning.

1. The first and least complex method of population projection is simple *extrapolation*. This can be done on an arithmetic basis, which involves equal amounts of change throughout each period, or on a geometric basis, which allows for constant rates of change.

2. The next possible technique is known as the *ratio method*, which attempts to relate the total population with some regularly measured variable, such as school enrollments, that is assumed to be constantly proportional to the total population.

3. The third approach, *correlation methods,* may be simple or multiple, and appears to be a somewhat more sophisticated variation of the ratio approach. Consequently, this approach tends to give better results, since the implied relationships can be measured and tested; however, there are some significant problems that can arise in using these techniques:

a. There is the possibility of omitting certain important variables even when using multiple regression.

b. Multicollinearity, in which the independent variables also are correlated with each other. The answer may be correct, but the effect attributed to each variable cannot be determined. This can be overcome, however, by the use of stepwise multiple regression.

c. Auto-correlation, in which the present value of the variable is related to earlier values of the same variable. This phenomenon can be dealt with by the use of difference equations.

d. Identification, in which case there are two curves—such as supply and demand—and either or both of these curves can shift so that neither can be identified by points of intersection between the stable curve and the moving curve. To overcome this, one of the curves must be made more variable than the other. This can be achieved by adding an extra independent variable to one equation. For example, weather could be added to agricultural supply, but not to demand. This would make the *supply* curve sufficiently variable to show how it moves along a rather stable *demand* curve.

e. There is spurious correlation or causality. Frequently, forecasting models are based upon a consistent relationship between variables without a consideration of the causes of the relationship. Such a situation can be very misleading as, for instance, a case in which academic salaries and the consumption of liquor are positively correlated. This can be avoided by using a structural model that is based upon a theoretical causal relationship rather than the simple outcome of mathematical manipulations.

4. The fourth approach to population forecasting that we will examine is the *component method*. This can be used for forecasting total population, or it can be used to measure the outcome for subgroups, which can be added together in order to arrive at the overall total. (For example, one might subdivide the population by age, sex, race, etc.) The component formula is rather simple and straightforward.

$P_{t+1} = P_t + B - D + M$, in which

P_{t+1} is the population after the completion of one period,
P_t is the population at the beginning of the period,
B is the number of births occurring during the period,
D is the number of deaths occurring during the period, and
M is the net migration during the period.

Using this method, the death rate is assumed to be constant. No one really looks for dramatic changes in mortality rates, since most major diseases have now been conquered; but this is true only if we are dealing with the overall population. There are possibilities of decreasing the mortality rate of specific subgroups, particularly infants and children. The birthrate is not so predictable; therefore, low, medium, and high fertility rates are used to generate a range of outcomes. The migration rate is very difficult to identify, and it often varies substantially from place to place. This migration rate can be estimated crudely by applying the formula $P_{t+1} - (P_t + B - D) + M$ to data acquired from previous censuses. This, of course, assumes that the data on births and deaths are accurate, and, unfortunately, such an assumption is seldom completely correct.

The preceding four population forecasting methods really do not meet the requirements for health planning population projections. A display of changes in individual cohorts[4] is needed in this area rather than simply assuming that the aggregate projections can be broken down into the same proportions as the base population. We know that each cohort has special population growth and health characteristics; therefore, we need to project by these subgroups. The projection should include adjustments for any changes of health status that may be likely to occur; for example, a survival rate for a given cohort may change as new health programs are added.

5. The *cohort survival method* will be the fifth and last approach to population forecasting that will be discussed here, since it appears to meet the criteria outlined above. Furthermore, the sum of the cohorts yields more accurate projections than do the aggregate projections described in our earlier approaches to population forecasting. Following are the steps to be used in the cohort survival method:

a. The population should be broken down into appropriate subgroups. The interval covered by each of the age groups should be equal to the periods of projection; for example, for 5-, 10-, or 20-year projections, use 5-year age groups (10–14, 45–49, etc.).

b. Multiply each subgroup by the appropriate survival rate. The survival rate is the complement of the death rate for the cohort. If the death rate is 10 per 10,000, the survival rate will be 9,990 per 10,000

c. Multiply female groups (in the 15 to 44 age group) by appropriate birthrates to get the number of births.

d. Multiply the total number of births by the proportion of male births and the proportion of female births to get the number of male and female births.

e. Multiply male and female births by the appropriate survival rates.

f. Add surviving births to the youngest cohorts.

g. Adjust each group for net migration.

h. Adjust each cohort for the percent who will advance to the next cohort due to age increase during the year.

[4] A cohort is a group of people with similar characteristics born in the same time period. All white women between 15 and 20 years of age is an example of a race-sex cohort.

In Figure 5, column t + 1 (cs) illustrates the computations by the cohort survival method. Note the following facts in the male cohort, in the 0–14 age group:

970 is the number of survivors out of the original 1,000,
70 is the number ($\frac{1}{14}$ of 1,000) that moved up to the 15–44 cohort, and
50 is the number of male babies that survived out of the 90 births to the 1,000 females in the 15–44 cohort.

This example ignores migration.

Column t + 1 (95.5%) illustrates the results that would have been obtained had the total population been decreasing at a rate of 4.5 percent over the past decade. The aggregate projection naturally would have been the same as the one obtained by the cohort survival, but when this aggregate is broken down into age groups on the basis of the age distribution at time t, it does not reveal the shifts in age and sex distribution, which are of critical importance in estimating health service requirements.

This concludes our review of Social Forecasting, wherein our concentration has been directed toward the quantitative approach—that is, projections of populations—rather than toward attitudes, values, and social systems.

TECHNOLOGICAL FORECASTING

Although some attempts at economic and demographic forecasting have been made by many health planning agencies and health institutions, few, if any, have explicitly entered the field of technological forecasting. This perhaps follows the tradition of classical economics, which treats technology as an exogenous variable included under the term *ceteris paribus*. Of course, as noted under economic forecasting, if no attempt is made to forecast, then there is an implicit assumption of no change. Such an assumption is clearly inappropriate in a modern, industrialized nation.

There are two basic approaches to technological forecasting. The first approach involves the prediction of a new or expanded application of an existing technology. For example, it is predicted that, by 1975, broadband communication systems and computer output on microfilms (COM) will make the transmission of X-ray data economically feasible; thus, medical centers could supply wide-ranging radiological services on a centralized

Age Group	Mortality Rate	Number		
		t	t + 1 (cs)	t + 1 (95.5%)
Male				
0–14	3%	1,000	970 − 70 + 50 = 950	955
15–44	1%	1,000	70 + 990 − 30 = 1,030	955
45–64	4%	1,000	30 + 960 − 50 = 940	955
65 and Over	22%	1,000	50 + 780 = 830	955
Total Male	8%	4,000	3,750	3,820
Female				
0–14	2%	1,000	980 − 80 + 40 = 940	955
15–44	0.5%	1,000	80 + 995 − 35 = 1,040	955
45–64	2%	1,000	35 + 980 − 50 = 965	955
65 and Over	11%	1,000	50 + 890 = 940	955
Total Female	4%	4,000	3,885	3,820
	Total	8,000	7,635	7,640

Natality rate = 9%
Male/female baby ratio: 55/45

Figure 5: Example of cohort survival and constant rate methods of population projections

basis. The second approach is to forecast a potential that does not now exist. For example, it might be forecast that by the year 2000 doctors will have acquired knowledge to prevent congenital defects. This would indicate a substantially lower number of mentally retarded needing care.

Generally, the health planner will not have the expertise necessary for making a technological forecast of this type. Rather, he must rely upon the knowledge, opinions, and judgments of those who are experts in the area of concern. It does not seem unreasonable, for example, that a hospital administrator should rely upon his radiologist to assist him in anticipating the types and uses of radiologic equipment during a period five years in the future when a new facility will be in operation; however, the radiologist's opinion alone is not sufficient basis for this type of forecast. To be meaningful, the prediction must also consider technical and economic feasibility, as well as acceptability to the users. Thus, we have a clear case in which some variation of the Delphi Technique, involving inputs from a variety of viewpoints, is most likely to yield a useful, valid forecast.

At this point, we will review the Delphi Technique, its relationship to forecasting in general, and how it can be used in technological forecasting in particular.

THE DELPHI TECHNIQUE[5]

Regardless of the approach taken to technological forecasting, the planner still faces the problem of advancing from the opinion of an individual to a more systematic forecast. One of the best-known techniques for achieving this end has been given the name "Delphi" by its developers, who are members of The RAND Corporation staff. As noted previously, this method, in its original form, probably exceeds the resources and requirements of most health planners; however, it can be readily adapted to meet the needs of almost any organization.

Briefly, the steps in this procedure are as follows: First, a panel of experts on a particular problem is drawn from both inside and outside the organization. Each expert is asked to make an anonymous forecast. Then, each panelist receives a composite feedback of the other panel members' answers. The feedback is designed to maintain the anonymity of each forecaster. Armed with this additional information, the experts then make a second round of forecasts. This process may be repeated three, four, or as many more times as necessary, until the decision maker is satisfied that the outcome is sufficiently refined.

By maintaining the anonymity of forecasters rather than assembling the experts together in face-to-face interaction, the decision maker allows the panelists more freedom to change their minds after reading other opinions. In a face-to-face session, they might be more concerned about defending their own forecast than in providing a good prediction.

In short, Delphi refines the judgments of experts. The first round of forecasts is not expected to produce a definitive answer. But, with successive rounds producing composite feedback, the answers to the initial problem gradually become more refined and improved and, coupled with the improved individual responses, add up to a better group judgment. Note particularly that the improvement results from giving each panelist the benefit of

---

[5] Helmer, Olaf. "Analysis of the Future. The Delphi Method." In: Bright, James R., ed. *Technological Forecasting for Industry and Government.* Englewood Cliffs, N.J., Prentice-Hall, 1968. pp. 116–122.

the other participants' knowledge, without allowing the participation of the other panel members to add social or emotional biases to their individual judgments.

Finally, it should be recognized that the use of the Delphi Technique need not be restricted to technological problems. It can be, and has been, successfully used to make forecasts in political and social areas; therefore, there is no reason to expect that it cannot be adapted for use in the health planning field should specific conditions warrant it.

SUMMARY

Since planning is for the future, the planner must have some method of estimating what the future will be like. His estimates are made explicit in a forecast that discusses not only what the future will be like, but also how that state was reached. The forecast must contain statements for political, social, economic, technological, and health components of the environment; however, it must be more than a set of projections. It must also stress the implications of those projections.

In this chapter, we discussed methods of providing the forecast for these components. For some, there are very specific techniques, based upon well-developed theories; however, even when such techniques are not available, there is at least one method—the Delphi Technique—which can be used to enhance materially the performance of expert forecasters. In many instances, the techniques described can be adopted directly, or they can be adapted by the health planner; in other cases, however, the technique in itself may exceed the resources available to him. Nevertheless, it is important that these methods be understood by the health planner so that he can judge the validity of forecasts provided by other agencies which have the capability of using these techniques.

REFERENCES

1. Atchley, Robert C. *Population Projections and Estimates for Local Areas.* Oxford, Ohio, Scripps Foundation, 1970.
2. Chambers, John C. et al. "How to Choose the Right Forecasting Technique." *Harvard Business Review, 49*(4):45–74, July–August 1971.

3. Ewald, William R., ed. *Environment and Policy: The Next Fifty Years.* Bloomington, Indiana University Press, 1968. pp. 59–110.
4. Laufman, Harold. "The Scientific Pressures." *Hospitals,* *45*(3):47–50, February 1, 1971.
5. Levin, L.S. "Building Toward the Future: Implications for Health Education." *American Journal of Public Health, 59*(11):1983–1991, November 1969.
6. Steiner, George A. *Top Management Planning.* New York, Macmillan, 1969. pp. 199–233.

CHAPTER 5

GOALS, POLICIES, AND OBJECTIVES

HIERARCHY

TYPES OF PLANNING

Planning encompasses a variety of types; this must be understood before the goals and objectives that relate to planning can be discussed intelligently. This fact was not recognized for a long time; therefore, until it became generally accepted, planners proceeded to make essentially the same projections, regardless of whether the undertaking called for short- or long-range planning. The results usually were disastrous, particularly in the long-range planning area. Eventually, however, planners began to perceive that long-range planning was different, and that long-range needs could not be dealt with in the same manner as short-term requirements. As a result, *normative planning* came into being.

Normative planning establishes goals, in contrast to technical planning, which deals with objectives. The relationship between goals and objectives is that *objectives*, essentially, are steps toward *goals*, and they are guided by *policies* that link goals and objectives. This is accomplished by setting forth the acceptable means that are to be used in working toward goals. Normative planning is sometimes called policy planning; in this perspective, it usually includes both goals and policies. Also, policy planning is sometimes used in lieu of specific master plans for the future, because the future is much too unpredictable for a single master plan. In contrast to a master plan, a policy plan provides flexibility, yet, at the same time, it ensures consistency and an ability to effect coordination.

The result of normative planning is a hierarchy of goals, policies, and objectives. In relation to the health care field, goals might be those end results toward which efforts are directed, such as improved health for the community; policies might be those courses of action undertaken to emphasize the prevention of disease rather than its cure; and objectives might be the establishment of such health-oriented programs as conducting periodic screening, providing immunization, or eliminating epidemics through health education. Therefore, we are progressing from the abstract to the concrete as we go from goals to objectives. Note, however, that the objectives just cited are not sufficiently concrete. We shall discuss this more fully later in this chapter.

OBJECTIVES

EFFECTS OF SETTING GOALS AND OBJECTIVES

In any undertaking—profit motivated or not—it should be observed that stated objectives can clarify the purpose of the organization. In some instances, these objectives can add new functions to fill gaps that were not previously recognized, and they may very well shift priorities among the functions. As a matter of fact, establishing priorities is often a more difficult task than stating the objectives themselves. The addition of new functions can, under certain circumstances, lead to a change in the organization itself, since it may point out that the original purpose of a service agency no longer exists. Finally, and perhaps of paramount importance, properly stated objectives will provide criteria for measuring the performance of any organization, and the health care field is no exception.

DEFINING OBJECTIVES

Measurability presents extremely difficult problems, because we are concerned with measuring output and not just input. We are concerned with changes in health per se and not just with activity in the health field; that is, activity is not necessarily productivity. An infinite number of man-hours might be committed to a program, but the results can be modest or even negligible. Thus, to be most useful, objectives should be measured by the results that they achieve rather than by input.

Here we encounter a problem in definition, because some things appear to be output when, in fact, they are simply intermediate input. For example, we recognize, in most cases, that physician man-hours are strictly input. On the other hand, although the visits that result from physician man-hours may seem to be output, actually they are not; they are simply intermediate inputs to the process of changing the health status of the population that is being served.

Another interesting aspect of defining objectives explicitly is that such definitions may show that the real problem is different from the one originally encountered. For example, a manpower shortage may not be the basic problem of the health care institution, but providing care is, and this problem may be solved by some other means than an approach that would increase the supply of manpower. Once the true objectives have been ascertained, we then have guides for the development of technical plans to achieve these objectives.

DEVELOPING OBJECTIVES

There are two approaches to developing objectives—general to specific and specific to general.[1] The first method moves from general to specific in six distinct steps:

1. Develop the current status of the organization.
2. Determine the current status of the organization's environment.
3. Project the status of the organization without any changes.
4. Develop a statement of the future environment.
5. Decide what the ideal situation for the organization should be in that future environment.
6. Contrast the idealized condition of step 5 to the static projection of step 3 to get realizable objectives for the organization, toward which each subunit must plan to work.

This process should be repeated on a periodic basis; an annual review may be sufficient to align the objectives with the changing environment. One must never be content, however, with objectives that were developed in the past. It is essential, first, that objectives be changed to keep abreast of the increased knowledge that accumulates as we approach the intended planning period; and, second, that these objectives go farther into the future to include periods not covered by previous planning cycles.

The alternative or reverse approach to the development of objectives—from specific to general—implies that, initially, planners are not capable of going through such a process; that is, people are simply unable to determine what their long-range objectives should be. Thus, the procedure is to begin with immediate problems and make very small plans to solve them. In so doing, people learn and are able to use their new knowledge to expand the

[1] Schaffer, Robert H. "Putting Action Into Planning." *Harvard Business Review*, 45(6):158–166, November–December 1967.

scope and time-frame of their planning effort so that eventually they are preparing long-range objectives as well.

The choice between these two methods depends to some extent upon a willingness to accept the ability of people to identify long-range goals that are relatively abstract and to translate such goals into meaningful short-term projects. Later in this chapter we will discuss various concepts of consumer knowledge, which will clarify the issues that are involved in choosing between the two approaches to developing objectives.

CRITERIA FOR GOOD OBJECTIVES

Regardless of the method used, to be acceptable and valid, the objectives must meet certain criteria.

1. Be within the authority of the agency or institution.
2. Be within the range of competence of the agency in terms of organization, personnel, techniques, equipment, and facilities.
3. Fit the time-frame available.
4. Be feasible within limits of the budget.
5. Be legal.
6. Fit the moral and value judgments of the community affected by the objective; for example, not all communities find abortion services an acceptable health care service.
7. Be practical; that is, they must be capable of being implemented.
8. Carry a minimum of unpleasant concomitants or side effects.
9. Be acceptable to whoever is responsible for carrying them out.
10. Be measurable.

The above list of criteria applies to any objective, regardless of the field of endeavor. Within the health field, however, the following generally accepted goals apply specifically to health services and should be used as additional criteria for evaluating objectives in this field. They must:

1. Be aimed at ensuring a healthful life, not merely caring for the sick.
2. Be available to all.
3. Be available at adequate levels.
4. Be accessible to all.
5. Assure timely action or receipt of services.
6. Be appropriate.

PARTICIPATION IN DETERMINATION OF OBJECTIVES

In regard to these latter criteria, many factors must be considered, including professional competence, effective utilization, and suitability to consumer culture; this has not been done in the past. A review of each of these factors follows.

Professional Competence: Frequently, consumer needs have been considered only to the extent that they were known and accepted by professionals as valid criteria for establishing objectives. Stated differently, expectations of consumer knowledge range from complete knowledge to complete ignorance. The latter is, perhaps, characteristic of the attitudes of many professionals. At one extreme, if the professional attitude of complete ignorance is accepted, there is the implicit assumption that the consumer simply does not know his own needs and, therefore, cannot evaluate the health services provided. At the other extreme, which accepts the idea of complete consumer knowledge, there is the implicit assumption that the individual is the best judge of his own welfare. Even though he cannot perform the services required, he does know when and how much service should be provided. For example, consider the issue of licensure. If we accept the consumer-knowledge idea, then we believe that licensure tends to create monopolies. If, however, we accept the consumer-ignorance idea, then we believe that licensure is necessary to protect the individual.

Turning to more general considerations, poor health seems to persist in certain neighborhoods despite the inauguration of many additional health care programs. This leads to the second factor to be considered, relating to consumer participation in determining objectives.

Effective Utilization: It is now generally accepted that poor health persists in some neighborhoods because the added resources are applied in a manner that is inappropriate to the situation. An unsuitable approach is usually directly attributable to a lack of understanding of the situation. Sociologists have clearly and frequently demonstrated that one group will generally see things quite differently than will other groups. Thus, it is natural—almost inevitable—that the optimal method of using the available resources, designed on the basis of the assumptions and biases of one group—that is, the providers—is less than ideal from the standpoint of the consumer. The resulting consumer dissatisfaction is clearly evident, even when the consumers belong to the same socioeconomic groups as the providers, but are not members of the providers' professional group. Surely, if there are disagreements and feelings of disenchantment between two groups that have many similarities, then certainly the likelihood of dissatisfaction will be far greater as differences between the two groups increase.

Dissatisfaction is equivalent to dislike, which leads to avoidance. Thus, services provided under a set of assumptions predicated on the benefits and desirability of medical care become even less appropriate when those services are used only in a crisis or on a last-resort basis. They are technically improper as well as culturally wrong, with the result that this use of resources tends to be ineffective even from the viewpoint of the professional designers of the system.

The obvious solution, therefore, is to decentralize control so that, within very broad limits, resources can be applied in the manner most appropriate to each situation. The need to do this has been recognized at all levels. For example, federal grants-in-aid for numerous, specific medical care programs have been replaced by single block grants that can be allocated in accordance with state priorities. This kind of action recognizes the fact that the health needs in Montana are probably quite different from those in New York. It is equally logical to recognize the difference between upstate New York and New York City and between Harlem and Washington Square.

This leads directly to the third factor, relating to consumer participation in determining objectives, that is, the adequacy of the consumers—in intellect, education, and experience.

Suitability to Consumer Culture: There are some who might cavil at the determination of health needs by lay persons. To do so is to confuse ends and means. The consumer well knows what the desired ends are and, as pointed out above, often has better insight into certain aspects of the means than does the professional. The insistence of the medical profession for maintaining the personalized doctor-patient relationship demonstrates that medical services cover a broad spectrum of activities ranging from totally technical to completely psychological. No one suggests that the consumer has the expertise to direct or make these selections on the technical end of the scale, but it is evident that he is the only one who truly knows the proper choices in terms of the social-psychological aspects of health care. In short, there are two kinds of expertise. They are not antithetical nor, in most cases, are they even conflicting. There will be a few cases at the margins where these areas of expertise meet, but the vast majority of situations clearly will be either on one side of this boundary or the other. The need then is to use the expertise that is available in both areas in a complementary fashion. This goal can be achieved if each group willingly accepts the contributions that can be made by the other.

To rephrase this slightly, there are five dimensions of medical care: adequacy, appropriateness, availability, accessibility, and acceptability. In the traditional health care system within this country, the first two of these dimensions have been adequately dealt with by the system of licensure and peer review. The latter three generally have been left to economic regulation by the mechanism of the free market, but this does not always work. Therefore, other mechanisms have been designed to provide for more effective input by the recipients of care, to give them meaningful control over these dimensions. Thus, we find that consumer councils of various types are now appearing in health institutions.

This consumer participation has led to many problems and misunderstandings. Often there is a definite difference in the degree of commitment perceived by the consumers and by the providers. For example, the provider of services may feel that he is using an optimum amount of resources to deal with a particular problem; on the other hand, the recipient of services may feel that the provider is merely shirking or slacking off, because the problem is not totally solved. Related to this is the consumers' distrust of providers, particularly by those who have had the experience of being used as guinea pigs or, euphemistically, as clinical material.

In contrast to this negative consumer feeling toward providers of health services is the problem of consumer involvement conflicting with the professionalism of the providers. A professional is defined as a person who is responsible for making decisions for other people which they are incapable of making for themselves. Thus, he has a fiduciary responsibility for providing health services; and any delegation or sharing of this responsibility leaves him subject to criticism for actions of which he is not in complete control.

Despite these and other problems that may arise, there are sufficient valid reasons to justify consumer participation in determining objectives. These reasons include the following factors: that participation will tend to reduce the alienation that exists between consumers and the institutions that are intended to serve them; that it will provide consumers with an opportunity to influence the decisions that affect them; that it will improve communication among all groups within the community; that it may provide socialization in the ways of the majority for minority groups (this perhaps is a debatable point); and, finally, that participation will tend to reinforce the underlying principles of our system of government. This final factor is sometimes difficult to accept, but it may be that the strengthening of democratic institutions is more important than the efficient delivery of health services.

Next is a discussion of how such consumer participation in determining objectives may be carried out in an effective manner.

CONDITIONS FOR EFFECTIVE PARTICIPATION

It is evident to those engaged in the health care field that participation will occur and will be maintained only if it is effective. There are certain conditions for effective participation that exist on both the consumer side and the provider side of the interaction. In the tabulation that follows, these conditions are outlined in a series of questions on resources, motivations, and structure.

RESOURCES

Consumer	*Provider*
Does the consumer have the intellectual and knowledge resources required to deal with the situation?	Is the provider dependent upon the consumer for resources, such as money and information?
Does the consumer have the material and economic resources required to participate effectively?	
Does the consumer have the social resources, including leadership, that are necessary for effective participation?	

MOTIVATION

Consumer	*Provider*
Do consumers believe that participation will be effective?	Do providers believe that consumers are potent?

Do consumers have relevant interests?

Do providers believe that consumer
participation is proper?

Do consumers feel that participation
is personally satisfying?

STRUCTURE

Consumer	*Provider*
Does the structure encourage partic-ipation rather than just permit it? For example, voting laws.	Is participation discretionary or mandatory? For example, P.L. 89–749 makes it mandatory, but on an advisory level.

COOPTATION VIS-A-VIS PARTICIPATION

Although consumer participation may be viewed as a means of achieving the ends described above, it may also be initiated for purposes of cooptation. Cooptation is the process of absorbing outside elements into the leadership or policy-determining structure of an organization as a means of averting threats to the organization's existence or stability. The need for cooptation arises when the formal authority, first, does not reflect the true balance of power; second, lacks historical legitimacy; or, third, is unable to mobilize the community for action.

Cooptation accomplishes the following: it establishes channels of communication; it allows the coopting agency to use the resources of coopted individuals and organizations; it provides knowledge, so that the broad policy can be implemented in accordance with local wishes and needs; and it shares responsibility, so that local citizens can be identified and committed to the agency and its program. In this last connection, it must be noted that cooptation does not necessarily guarantee an effective voice in the decision-making process. Consequently, the coopted may be sharing responsibility for activities over which they had virtually no control. It must be borne in mind, however, that this often works both ways; therefore, although the coopter may influence the coopted, very often the coopted can seize effective control of the organization.

In any event, for an organization to survive, it must seek the support of those people within the community who have power resources, such as wealth, status in formal organizations, expertise, political popularity, and capability to effect symbolic manipulation; for example, TV stations, newspapers, etc. Every member of a community has some of these resources, but, obviously, they are not equally distributed.

It is necessary, therefore, to identify the people in the community who are in a position to bring an adequate amount of these resources to the organization in order to ensure its effectiveness. How can these people be identified? There are a number of theories about the power structure within a community, although the one which is probably best-known is the elitist theory.

The Elitist Theory: This theory was developed by sociologists and achieved its widest publicity from a study done by Floyd Hunter in Atlanta, Georgia.[2] It posits a situation whereby all policy is made covertly by a ruling clique of economic influentials; in turn, the programs effecting these policies are implemented by a core of professionals who are, for all practical purposes, subservient to the ruling group. It should be noted, however, that Hunter's study—on which this theory is based—employed the so-called reputational method; the investigator asked a number of people in the community who the influentials were and then narrowed this field down to a relatively small number from those whose names appeared repeatedly on the responses.

Theory of the Pluralists: A second common theory concerning the community power structure is that of the pluralists. Their position was popularized by Robert Dahl's study in New Haven, Connecticut.[3] This study found that there had been a shift over time from the elite situation, described by Hunter, to one in which there was a variety of decision-making groups, and that the decision-making power shifted from issue to issue. This concept was based upon a different methodology, which involved two approaches—the positional and the decisional. In the positional approach, one simply looks to see which people fill formal organizational roles within a community, for example, a mayor. In the decisional method, one must do historical research to discover which people in the community were influential in arriving at certain major decisions.

An important point to note is that the difference between Dahl's theory (pluralistic) and Hunter's theory (elitist) is not one between a monolithic, elite group and popular democracy, but rather between a monolithic, elite

---

[2] Hunter, Floyd. *Community Power Structure.* Chapel Hill, N.C., University of North Carolina Press, 1953.
[3] Dahl, Robert A. *Who Governs.* New Haven, Conn., Yale University Press, 1962.

group and pluralistic group decision making. In the latter case, the decision makers on any issue again are a small group who possess the necessary power resources; but it must be assumed that the composition of the decision-making group probably changes dramatically from one issue to another.

One of the major criticisms of both these studies, of course, was that they overlooked the importance of negative decisions; both methodologies neglected to consider the power of certain individuals to prevent an action from happening and reported only those cases in which some positive action was taken.

Other Power Structure Theories: Later studies by Presthus[4] and others, such as Kammerer,[5] suggest that, in fact, there is a continuum of power structure types. As the community grows, it moves along this continuum from the monolithic situation or monopoly of power described by Hunter to the diffuse competitive structure described by Dahl. Banfield's study of Chicago[6] asserts that the single elite group cannot exist because there would be no means of communication among them on the scale required for an area of that size; furthermore, that the diversity of interests among the people possessing the power resources in such a community would eventually lead, first, to conflict and, then, to dissolution of the monolithic group.

A practical application of these theories is demonstrated in Wilson's study,[7] which was made when a variety of communities throughout the country were attempting to assess their health status. In this study, he used all three methods: the reputational method, the decision method, and the positional method. His findings were rather interesting. First, most community leaders do not see health as a major problem. This may have changed since the mid-1960's, but, if one looks at certain communities today, there still is reason to suspect that this may be true. Second, the leaders tend to be content with the status quo and seek to avoid conflicts which may affect their own status or power. Third, economic leaders tend to dominate any affair that involves money, whereas political leaders are strong where legislation and regulation are necessary. But the political leaders tend to avoid health matters, since there seems to be little payoff to them in terms of increasing

[4] Presthus, Robert V. *Men at the Top.* New York, Oxford University Press, 1964.
[5] Kammerer, Gladys M. *The Urban Political Community: Profiles in Town Politics.* Boston, Houghton Mifflin, 1963.
[6] Banfield, Edward C. *Political Influence.* New York, Free Press, 1961.
[7] Wilson, Robert N. *Community Structure and Health Action.* Washington, D.C., Public Affairs Press, 1968. pp. 28–35, 46, 58, 61–69, 76–97.

their resources through political influence. Finally, Wilson discovered that professionals seem to have influence only in very narrow technical areas, such as fluoridation.

For the practicing health administrator or health planner, there are certain implications in all these studies. The first is one of identification: from a practical point of operation, the planner must identify the people who can provide meaningful community participation in his endeavors. These people can be identified by the use of three methods—reputational, decisional, and positional. These methods can be combined without too much difficulty over a relatively short period of time; that is, when a health planner arrives in a community with which he is unfamiliar, the astute use of these methods will help him assay the health situation. For example, it is relatively easy to obtain past copies of newspapers in order to discover what the health issues have been and who has been involved, thereby using the decisional method. It is equally easy to discover past and present holders of key positions within the community; that is, positioning the people. Finally, informal conversations without an elaborate survey will identify rather quickly those people who have the reputation of being influential in the health field; thus, a practical application can be made of the reputational method.

Another implication suggested by these studies is that the health administrator may experience considerable difficulty in motivating the obvious community leaders to use their power in the health field. Power is a scarce resource and, as with any scarce resource, the possessor is generally unwilling to invest it unless he can foresee an adequate return on his investment.

Finally, it would appear from these studies that a variety of incentives will be necessary to motivate the different types of leaders who will be required to participate if the health administrator or planner intends to cover all the areas that are involved in a comprehensive health scheme.

REFERENCES

1. American Society of Planning Officials. *Planning 1968*. Chicago, 1968. pp. 33–46.
2. Cadmus, Robert R. et al. "Community Concern, Hospital Interest." *Modern Hospital, 113*(2):78–98, August 1969.
3. Cathcart, H. Robert. "Reaching the Unreachables." *Hospitals, 45*(19):37–40, October 1, 1971.

4. Colt, Avery M. "Public Policy and Planning Criteria in Public Health." *American Journal of Public Health, 59*(9):1678–1685, September 1969.

5. Hochbaum, G.M. "Consumer Participation in Health Planning: Toward Conceptual Clarification." *American Journal of Public Health, 59*(9): 1698–1705, September 1969.

6. O'Donnell, Edward J. and Chilman, Catherine S. "Poor People on Public Welfare Boards and Committees; Participation in Policy-Making?" *Welfare in Review, 7*(3):1–10, May 1969.

7. Ross, M.H. "Transition in Hospital Programs." *Hospitals, 43*(24):49–53, December 16, 1969.

8. Zborowski, Mark. "The Changing Urban Scene." *Hospitals, 44*(23): 33–36, December 1, 1970.

CHAPTER 6

SPATIAL ASPECTS OF HEALTH PLANNING

The health planner must concern himself with two types of spatial considerations—area and location. In terms of area, quite frequently a health service is aimed at a specific geographic domain, in which instance the planner's problem becomes one of definition—of both boundaries and the area within those boundaries. The second consideration is where to locate the service being planned for the area. Typically, we think of either a fixed site or several sites. This is true whether the area to be served has firm geographic boundaries or whether it comprises an entire population. There are a few instances, however, when the planner is concerned with location of a slightly different nature, as when services are offered on a mobile basis to a fixed population. In either case, however, the need for making decisions on the basis of spatial considerations still remains.

SOCIOECONOMIC AND DEMOGRAPHIC FACTORS AFFECTING DEMAND

There are a number of reasons for being concerned with spatial relationships, but here the discussion will be directed toward identifying the socioeconomic and demographic factors that affect demand for health services, both directly and indirectly. Factors that will be examined here will include those that relate to the character of the population, the concept of regionalization, the availability of health services, and others; also, those factors that relate to the transportation of clients to and from these health services, the accessibility of the services, and other environmental factors.

First, concerning those factors that relate to the character of the population, the concept of regionalization, the availability of complementary services, and the market areas affecting demand:

1. The health planner must know the character of the population within the area to be served, in order to determine the probable interaction between population (given its social, cultural, and ethnic characteristics), and the rules and sponsorship of the health services being offered. For example, it is relatively easy to point out numerous cases in which services are technically available, although there may be both economic and religious barriers to the use of these services.

2. Health planners must be concerned with duplication of services within the areas defined.

3. Regionalization must be considered. Regionalization is an important concept, since it can effect economies of scale; however, it requires a minimum population in order to be viable, and, of course, the population minimum varies with the type of service. Regionalization will be discussed more fully later in this section.

4. Economies of scale can be offset by transportation costs relating to five distinct groups: professional providers, nonprofessional employees, inpatients, outpatients, and visitors. For example, regionalization of specialized pediatric services may seem feasible from the standpoint of economies of scale, but considering the unusually high requirement for frequent visits by the family, which might result in the absence of parents from a home where there are other children, it becomes evident that the regionalization concept will impose particularly high costs upon this group.

5. The health planner must determine the availability of complementary services that would increase the use of a planned facility; for example, a clinic might be located adjacent to a shopping center.

6. Finally, the health planner must look at market areas, since it has been proven that familiarity tends to make distances psychologically shorter; that is, if there are two trips of the same distance, the one that has been made frequently will seem much shorter than the one which is new and unfamiliar.

Next, let us study the factors that affect demand indirectly. Here, the planner must consider what is involved in transporting patients between their homes and the location of services. It appears that patients are indifferent to distances of up to about two miles when they are considering hospital services; however, it is also quite clear that convenience to health services can influence utilization. For example, in the past, persons who have studied this situation have said that hospitals should be no more than 50 miles away from a population center, with 100 miles between hospitals. At that time—during the early days of Hill-Burton—the major concern was with the location of rural facilities. As a rule of thumb, perhaps this concept was not too bad; however, it certainly overlooked many complexities, such as natural barriers.

Another factor is utilization of facilities. In an urban area, this problem tends toward overuse of convenient facilities and underuse of others. This raises two issues: First, what is the normal capacity or the optimum utilization of a particular facility? Second, what are the costs of suboptimization? Both overuse and underuse result in excessive costs. It is obvious that fixed operating costs for unfilled hospital beds represent a cost to the community. It is less obvious, but equally true, that overutilization of a facility also can result in very high costs because premiums must be paid to provide the excess services. For example, overtime at a premium rate may have to be paid to members of the hospital staff in order to provide adequate service to patients when a hospital is occupied at 100 percent.

In short, some of the most crucial factors concerning location and utilization of facilities include space, accessibility, transportation, communications, and environment. All of these are interrelated to some extent. For example, when considering expansion of a hospital, administrators must be concerned not only with having enough space to expand the facility itself, which frequently can be accomplished by building upward on the existing facility, but they also must be concerned with the subsequent increased use of the facility, which will create, among other considerations, the need for substantially more parking spaces. Many administrators, to their chagrin, have discovered that inadequate planning for parking spaces has been very costly in terms of acrimonious relations with the surrounding community.

Other environmental factors also must be kept in mind; for example, it would be absurd to establish a prenatal clinic in an industrial area. Health planning, of course, is not concerned only with personal health problems; the health planner also must consider the broader area covered by environmental problems. This creates a very difficult task for the health planner—the identification of environmental problem sheds. For example, the problem shed for water pollution in the Metropolitan Washington, D.C. area includes several states and several hundred miles of the Potomac River. There also are epidemiological considerations, since diseases often are affected by a wide variety of ecological factors including temperature, rainfall, agricultural practices, and population densities of various plants, insects, and animals. These factors tend to produce geographic disease patterns, for example, where agricultural practices still involve the use of human excrement for fertilizer.

Finally, there are many spatial factors that indirectly affect the availability of resources. For example, certain rural communities and urban areas are considered unattractive by professional workers, and thus are medically underserved. A critical resource is funds, and frequently there are distinct differences among geographic areas in the availability of funds. The most obvious example of this is evident in the relatively affluent and strong tax-base areas of the suburbs, which have a relatively low demand for public services, as compared to the high demand for public services in the central city, where usually there is a very weak and distinctly limited tax base upon which the city can draw.

COMMUNITY DETERMINATION

Clearly, the identification of a health service community is not a simple matter. A useful attempt to address this issue was "The Community of Solution,"[1] made by the National Commission on Community Health Services. The Community of Solution is not just a geographic concept to be determined by plane geometry; it tends to be a combination of the following seven subcommunities:

Community of Identifiable Need: An identifiable need is based on a factually substantiated "lack"—that is, the absence of something needed—which the overall organized society feels is both correctable and deserving of attention. A community of identifiable need is the group itself that is in need. Usually, the community of need is bounded by a limited, geographically definable area; however, it may be a specific population group, such as migrant workers, who are a group without a fixed geographic location.

Community of Problem Ecology: Some problems have a clearly defined set of boundaries, since the causal agent exists only within a well-established and specified terrain. Where systems analysis of a condition or a disease indicates that there are relevant geographic, social, or other boundaries to its

---

1 National Commission on Community Health Services. *Health Is a Community Affair.* Cambridge, Mass., Harvard University Press, 1966. pp. 2–9.

occurrence, these boundaries become significant for planning. In some instances, planning will have to embrace the entire nation; but, more often, it is possible to define a subregion within which effective action can be taken. It is important to note, however, that for some kinds of problems, particularly those of an environmental nature, the region becomes quite large. Returning to the previous example of water pollution in Washington, D.C., it should be noted that any attempt to cleanse only that part of the Potomac River that is bounded by the city itself would be virtually futile.

Community of Concern: This may cover a much larger area than merely that area where the problem occurs, because of "spill-over effects." Poor health in a ghetto area, for example, tends to raise taxes for nonghetto residents. Also, poor health in such an area can lead to the spread of communicable diseases into other, more affluent areas. Thus, the affluent areas are a part of the community of concern.

Community of Special Interest: This community seldom has specific geographic boundaries. Rather it tends to be comprised of groups of people, regardless of origin, who have common interests. A typical example would be a group of professionals and charitable associations, all of whom are interested in eradicating some specific illness, such as glaucoma or emphysema.

Community of Viability: This is the community that can support the planned activity; therefore, it must have enough clients to make the activity feasible. Thus, a viable community for open heart surgery will differ significantly from the viable community for a smallpox vaccination program.

Community of Resources: This is the area wherein resources can be found to do the particular job. Obviously, there is no guarantee that the distribution of a problem and the distribution of the resources needed to solve the particular problem will be identical or even similar.

Community of Action Capability: This is the group of people who may, and often do, have the potential for taking effective action to correct the problems identified. Frequently, because of legal and financial considerations, this community must be defined in terms of political subdivisions. There are occasions, however, when groups can operate effectively without respect to political boundaries; for example, voluntary health agencies or, on occasion, political subdivisions united into a common organization, such as a council of governments.

It is evident that the Community of Solution, defined through an analysis of these seven factors, in most cases will be an ill-defined, multidimensional entity. Conceptually, this is not unappealing; however, as a practical matter, it often happens that we must deal in terms of political jurisdictions. The Advisory Commission on Intergovernmental Relations (ACIR) has addressed this issue from that viewpoint and has developed an extremely useful set of guidelines for determining the proper assignment of responsibility for the performance of urban functions.[2] The ACIR, however, is addressing this issue from the public administration point of view which, in turn, concerns itself with such things as the establishment of local jurisdictions (for example, special districts) and the distribution of functions among county, state, city, township, and other governmental entities. Although the initial ACIR analysis dealt primarily with traditional public health services, it is quite clear that the model is applicable to all types of health services. Their criteria are as follows:

1. The jurisdiction should be large enough so that most benefits can be realized within its bounds, which means that different functions must necessarily be assigned to different levels of government. For example, a medical school might be assigned to the state government, while direct, personal health services could be assigned to a local governmental agency.
2. The area of jurisdiction must be large enough to permit realization of economies of scale.
3. The geographic area must be adequate for effective performance. Returning again to the water pollution example, the watershed must contain the source of the water as well as the users.
4. The unit of government must have both the legal and administrative ability to carry out the activities. This, incidentally, includes the ability to finance them. It should be noted, however, that local jurisdictions in our form of government are allowed to perform only those functions that have been expressly delegated to them by the state, because it is within the state government that all residual powers reside. Thus, if a local jurisdiction

[2] Advisory Commission on Intergovernmental Relations. *Performance of Urban Functions: Local and Areawide.* Washington, D.C., U.S. Government Printing Office, 1963.

wants to begin a new activity that is not in its charter, it must receive prior approval from the state—usually in the form of an amendment to its charter—before it can undertake such an activity.

5. A sufficient number of functions must be included in this local jurisdiction so that conflicting interests can be considered and balanced within the one unit of government. This criterion is intended to avoid unilateral decision making and to emphasize the need for coordinating the many services provided by government.

6. The performance of the function must be accessible to, and controllable by, the residents of the local jurisdiction. This is another version of the emphasis that is placed on consumer participation. What we need is a balance between the economies of scale, the spread of authority, etc., and closeness to the people. Frequently, some economies and efficiency are sacrificed to gain a more meaningful democratic process; however, this is not to suggest that we should go to the extreme of establishing a multitude of small units. In general, people can participate far more effectively in one large, multipurpose government that is highly visible than in a welter of small, overlapping special governments, which is a condition typical in many suburbs.

REGIONALIZATION

Regionalization is a term frequently used to describe the implementation of the above concepts.

A region is a geographic area containing a set of homogeneous people, things, and circumstances. It is generally assumed that a region is an optimal territorial unit for coordinated economic and/or social planning. Usually, a region has a center, plus outlying areas. The center may not be physically at the midpoint of the area, but it does represent a concentration of strength in contrast to the relative weakness of the outlying areas. The region must be defined further as a system of exchanges between the center and the outlying areas. This concept is illustrated by the Rourke[3] approach to service area definition. Rourke proposes a central, sophisticated medical complex to which patients can be referred from peripheral and base service hospitals.

---

[3] Frieden, Bernard J. and Peters, James. "Urban Planning and Health Services: Opportunities for Cooperation." *Journal of the American Institute of Planners, 36*(2):90, March 1970.

As long ago as 1932, the Committee on the Costs of Medical Care urged the integration of primary and specialized care through regionalization. The Hill-Burton program was intended to develop better regional distribution of health facilities, but it contained no mechanism for establishing a system of interaction among the facilities. The Regional Medical Program has attempted to correct this deficiency.[4]

The linkages which evolve, however, are contingent upon the allocation of resources. For example, a rural hospital will establish referral patterns with an urban medical center only for those specialities in which its own staff lacks competence. Unfortunately, there is no overall resource for allocating authority, other than the imperfect market mechanism; consequently, activities are often decentralized to a level where economies of scale are lost. Effective regionalization requires some degree of centralized authority. In general, this component is lacking in Regional Medical Programs. To some extent, this is attributable to the concessions that were made to the American Medical Association while the De Bakey Commission's recommendations were being translated into P.L. 89–239, but the role of the Department of Health, Education, and Welfare in implementing the law cannot be ignored as another causative agent. The apparent willingness of the Federal Government to accept and fund virtually any cooperative venture, no matter how tenuous the linkages, has done much to vitiate this aspect of RMP.[5]

There are many reasons why the original, strong concept of regionalization has been opposed. First, small institutions fear the medical schools which, typically, occupy the central location of any health region. Second, transferring patients is discouraged because of the economic losses incurred by the transferrer—hospital and/or physician. Third, centralization of specialized services tends to put severe limitations on the growth and prestige of institutions in outlying areas. Fourth, patients expect to be treated within their own community. This fourth factor—emphasis on accessibility at the expense of efficiency—reinforces the drive of outlying institutions to expand even when there is little prospect that they will ever attain full utilization of the additional services or facilities.

These factors have tended to reinforce the traditional use of service areas as a key concept in health planning.

4 Bodenheimer, Thomas S., M.D. "Regional Medical Programs: No Road to Regionalization." *Medical Care Review,* 26(11):1127, December 1969.
5 *Ibid.,* pp. 1133–35.

SERVICE AREAS

Historically, health service planning has been based upon a concept of service areas. This is particularly true in the case of facilities planning. In fact, many approaches are overly simplified attempts to define a health services community based only on a few dimensions. The following examples serve to explain the concept of service areas:

1. First, there is the service area approach suggested by McGibony,[6] which involves seven steps: plot the location of existing facilities on a map; outline tentative service areas based on political boundaries and distances; check travel flow based on highways; check for physical barriers to travel, for example, the Anacostia River in the District of Columbia; determine existing trade areas; check the use patterns of other health facilities (residences of patients may be obtained from hospital records, but often this is inadequate; location of doctors' offices also must be considered since it is the doctor who typically directs the patient to a hospital); and determine the characteristics of population, including age, income level, racial composition, ethnic groups, etc. Unfortunately, no rules are provided for the use of these data once they have been collected, except to apply them in a commonsense manner.

2. In mental health planning, the concept of a catchment area has evolved. Since there is no universal definition of a community, the mental health authorities adopted a range of population size—namely, from 75,000 to 200,000. This presumes that everyone in the area has easy access to the facilities. It ignores political boundaries, and it assumes that the mental health problems are fairly evenly distributed among all population groups. Because of the looseness of this definition, it has been applied in a variety of ways. For example, Illinois bases its catchment area on the distance from the mental health hospital. Pennsylvania's catchment area conforms strictly to county boundaries. In Arizona, it is based on geographic area and distance from a mental health center. Problems encountered in using the catchment area concept are numerous. Census data are based on political boundaries; thus, it becomes very difficult to determine the boundaries of a population-based catchment area. Population

---

[6] McGibony, John R., M.D. *Principles of Hospital Administration.* New York, G. P. Putnam's Sons, 1969. p. 29.

shifts, of course, require an adjustment of boundaries. Also, there is the unanswered question of what should be done when the population is very sparse or very dense. For example, 75,000 people could be spread so widely that one community mental health center would not be accessible to everyone within the catchment area.

3. A third and somewhat different approach to the service area problem is that taken by Anthony Rourke in one of his Nebraska studies. In this case, he proposed three service areas and defined them on the basis of patient origin data. The first was called a base service area, and in it would be placed those hospitals that could serve most of the medical needs of their patients. In the second or peripheral service area would be found those hospitals which would serve, first, as a base service area, but, more importantly, would provide some of the more sophisticated services that were not available in those hospitals designated as base service area institutions. Finally, there would be the regional service area. This would concentrate on those hospitals which, to some extent, would be used for base and peripheral services, but primarily would focus upon providing highly specialized services for persons normally treated at other base and peripheral service hospitals.

4. Still another approach to the service area concept was adopted in a hospital study in Cleveland. In this particular case, census tracts were designated service areas and were allocated to various institutions on the basis of the proportion of patients served from any one census tract. Thus, if there were four hospitals that received patients from a single census tract, then the responsibility for that entire census tract would be assigned to whichever hospital received the highest proportion of the patients. Obviously, this is inaccurate methodology.

5. The patient flow matrix proposed by Morrill and Earickson[7] is a much more sophisticated approach. It assumes that use of the nearest hospital is an ideal and then measures the deviations from this ideal. Their Chicago study clearly shows, first, that the service area, as normally defined, is a gross misrepresentation of the facts. For example, 35 to 40 percent of all patients crossed boundaries. Second, service areas cut across normal community boundaries, thus making a population forecast nearly impossible. It is interesting to observe that, with recent developments in small-area data from the 1970 Census, it should be possible to do a much better job of

[7] Morrill, Richard L. and Earickson, Robert. "Locational Efficiency of Chicago Hospitals: An Experimental Model." *Health Services Research*, 4(2):128–141, Summer 1969.

defining service areas on the basis of patient origin. Not too many communities, however, have the geographic base file that is necessary to convert ordinary maps into locational grids and then to plot residential addresses on these grids.

6. Another approach to service area definition is that proposed by a George Washington University Health Care Administration alumnus, Dorn K. Johnstone, in his Major Report.[8] His concept is based on the assumption that service areas should be determined by the hospital alone. Rather than planning for the community, his methodology involves the hospital in a planning program for itself. Johnstone's notion may be controversial, however, his manner of computation is interesting.

Johnstone's method distinguishes between two types of service areas: the primary medical service area and a larger geographic area for more highly specialized services.

The first—the medical service area—is the one for which most institutions will carry out the bulk of their planning effort. Here, the hospital presumably is the organizational focal point for all health services. In this respect, it is similar to the type of hospital described by Rourke as a base service hospital. The second—the geographic area—is similar to that served by a regional or peripheral hospital. Presumably, here, there is some combination of the two, and, judging from Johnstone's descriptions, it would appear to be legitimate to consider his second service area as a combination of Rourke's regional and peripheral service areas.

By reversing the requirements approach, in which a given population is multiplied by some standard factor in order to determine the necessary number of beds, Johnstone assumes a number of beds and then determines how many people the hospital can serve. Thus, instead of saying that Beds are equal to Population times a Ratio ($B = P \times R$), Johnstone's formula would be Population equals Beds divided by Ratio ($P = B \div R$), or, the population that can be served is equal to the number of beds divided by the ratio of beds to population. For example, if there is a 200-bed hospital and a requirement ratio of 4 beds per 1,000 people, then it may be presumed that the hospital can serve about 50,000 people. Johnstone, however, recognizes that this is not totally realistic, and therefore proceeds

8 Johnstone, Dorn K. "The Concept and Definition of an Individual Hospital Geographic Service Area." Major Report Submitted to the Faculty of the Department of Health Care Administration of the School of Government and Business Administration of the George Washington University, January 1971.

to modify the concept by proposing two constraints which he entitles the *index of relevance* and the *index of commitment*.

His index of relevance recognizes that not everyone in a given community will use a single facility; thus, he determines relevance by dividing the average daily census from a selected community in hospital A by the total average daily census in all hospitals. For example, if, on the average, 50 people in a given area are patients in all hospitals, and 25 of these are patients in the hospital with which we are concerned, then the index of relevance for the hospital is .5 or R (Relevance) = 25/50. This relevance factor is included in the basic formula as a multiplier of the denominator. Thus, Population equals Beds divided by the product of the Utilization factor multiplied by the Relevance factor: that is, $P = B \div (U \times R)$; or, returning to our earlier example, $P = (200 \div (4 \times .5)) \times 1,000$, which is equal to 100,000 people. Applying the index of relevance has the effect of increasing the population size that can be served by the hospital with which we are concerned. It should also be apparent by examining the formula that the population size of the geographic service area varies inversely with the hospital's index of relevance.

Johnstone's index of commitment recognizes the fact that, particularly in specialty hospitals, only a portion of the hospital bed complement can be allocated for the purpose of delivering health services to a specifically defined community of people. For example, in the regional hospital, some portion of the total number of beds would be allocated for base service needs, while the remainder of the beds would be reserved for the specialty needs of the region. The index of commitment determines what portion will be allocated to base services and how much of the hospital's capacity will be reserved for specialty services in its role as a regional or peripheral service area hospital.

The hospital may choose to designate a commitment level arbitrarily, or it may wish to determine its index of commitment from experience. To make this computation on the basis of current practice, the hospital must divide the average daily census of its base service area by the total average daily hospital census. For example, if a hospital has an average daily census of 250 patients, 100 of whom reside within the base service area, then its index of commitment for that area is .4; that is, C (Commitment) = 100/250. This commitment factor is applied to the total number of beds available in the original formula in order to determine the population size, as follows: Population equals (number of Beds times index of Commitment) divided by (ratio of Beds to Population times index of Relevance); or, in symbols, $P = (BC) \div (UR)$. It should be noted that the application of the commitment factor reduces the population size of the hospital's base service area; that is, the population size of the geographic service area varies directly with the hospital's index of commitment.

Clearly, Johnstone's index of commitment and index of relevance work in opposite directions, thus tending to offset one another. Therefore, if there is a hospital with 200 beds, an index of commitment of .4, a bed ratio of 4 beds per 1,000 people, and an index of relevance of .5, a population of 40,000 persons could be served; specifically, the formula would read: $P = ((200 \times .4) \div (4 \times .5)) \times 1,000 = 40,000$. Perhaps the most important thing to be learned from Johnstone's approach is that it identifies the significance of decisions that are made by the hospital administration in terms of their effect upon its ability to provide community services.

This concludes our series of examples explaining the service area concept. As a practical matter, this concept is widely accepted and has many strong advocates. In actual practice, it is based upon political boundaries, assignment of areas to hospitals which serve a majority of patients, and the realities of resources allocation. Here, we often find a certain amount of gerrymandering in order to justify the need to build more beds. Unfortunately, many of the weaknesses of the service area concept are not widely recognized. For example, it makes heroic assumptions that the service areas are mutually exclusive. This assumption is invalidated for hospitals (but not necessarily for other medical facilities, such as nursing homes) by a number of factors. These include transportation accessibility, economic accessibility, the reputation of the institution, formal and informal referral patterns, and ethnic and religious ties. The Chicago study previously cited clearly shows the impact these factors can have upon hospital utilization.

LOCATIONAL MODELS

Since the service area has weaknesses, Schneider[9] has proposed the alternative of allocating beds on a community-wide basis and treating location as a

---

[9] Schneider, J.B. "New Approach to Areawide Planning of Metropolitan Hospital Systems." *Hospitals,* 42(8):79–83, April 16, 1968.

secondary question. He offers a spatial model based on distribution of patients and on distance from hospitals; however, his model also has many serious limitations. First, hospitals do not necessarily offer the same kinds of services. Second, all patients do not have equal access to all hospitals. In addition to the distance factor, with which Schneider deals, there are economic, psychological, and geographic barriers. Regarding the last, Schneider's study was made for Cincinnati, Ohio, and he either overlooked, or chose to ignore, the fact that the Ohio River, which separates Cincinnati from the suburban area located in Kentucky, prevents a substantial number of people from coming to Cincinnati hospitals.

Since Schneider developed this model several years ago, there have been a number of more sophisticated attempts to cope with some of these problems. One of the most recent is the work by Martin Baum,[10] who has developed a simulation model that allows for the placement of services in three types of facilities: a hospital, a neighborhood health center, or a storefront clinic. Actually, the model can deal with any conceivable combination of these service placements. Having made an initial allocation, the model is then run to determine the costs—both cost of resource allocations and cost to the clientele using the facilities. The cost to clientele is measured by such things as travel time and waiting time. The resource costs are affected by the degree of decentralization. The model computes the utilization time of resources. Currently, the costs of resources are computed outside the basic model, since this is a matter of simple arithmetic. After the initial run has been made, and base-line data has been developed, it is then possible to vary the location of the three types of facilities. This is done in an attempt to improve patient costs and/or to vary the facilities at which the various services are offered so that trade-offs can be made between costs of resources used and costs to clientele using those resources.

SITE FACTORS

Finally, when the approximate location in which a facility should be placed has been identified, attention must be given to the variety of factors that will determine the desirability of such location. First, there are the site fac-

10 Baum, Martin A. "A Model for the Examination of Urban Primary Care Health Delivery Systems with Special Emphasis on the Poor." Unpublished Ph.D. Dissertion. Washington, D.C., American University, September 1971.

tors, including room for expansion, parking, and the availability of services. A service of considerable importance to health facilities, particularly inpatient facilities, is a fire department. Second, there are the accessibility factors, involving transportation systems and roads, distance from patients, and terrain barriers such as rivers and mountains. Finally, neighborhood characteristics will have a great bearing upon the desirability of the site. These include the current land use, renewal plans, existence of related facilities such as nursing homes, and nuisance factors—noise, odor, smoke, or dust.

CHAPTER *7*

COMMUNITY CHARACTERISTICS
AND RESOURCES

The Community of Solution is not just a geographic area determined by plane geometry, but, rather, it might be a combination of nonplace geographic entities comprising many interrelating subcommunities of problem ecology, concern, special interest, viability, action, capability, resources, and political jurisdictions.

To best describe the characteristics of a community, one must begin by determining what constitutes these characteristics. First, there are the demographic characteristics, which might be called the anatomy of a community; then, there are the ecologic characteristics, which might be termed the community's physiology; and, finally, there is the health status of the community, which might be called its symptomatology. The following discussion will deal with all three of these community characteristics and the several factors relating to each.

DEMOGRAPHIC CHARACTERISTICS

The population size (that is, the total number of people) provides an estimate of the workload for which the planning or programming is being carried out. The population, of course, can be grouped by such characteristics as age and sex distribution; but population size must be adjusted whenever changes occur as a result of fertility and natality, mortality, and in- and out-migration.

As has been implied, population size alone is inadequate for estimating health requirements; therefore, other characteristics must be considered, such as sex ratio, age distribution, population factors involving substantial urban-rural or regional differences, ethnic and cultural differences and religion, economic status, marital status, education, and urban pathology (such as crime). These are explained briefly below:

Sex ratio has a direct affect upon marriage and birth rates and upon family patterns; indirectly, it affects occupational patterns and longevity.

Age distribution affects the patterns of mortality and morbidity, which vary considerably with different age groups; in addition, it affects the rates of disability caused by acute and chronic diseases. Mortality rates and the causes of death are different for each age group. The same is true for morbidity and disability rates.

Population density affects the level of services as well as living conditions. Population migration affects the rate of growth in different areas of the community.

Ethnic and cultural characteristics and variations can influence the outlook toward utilization of health care services, as can *religious beliefs* and teachings.

Economic status affects a population's ability to procure and utilize health services and to maintain healthful standards of living.

Differences in *marital status* may affect such things as the birth rate, divorce rate, and the ability to provide home health and other services.

Level of *education* affects utilization of health services and, in particular, influences approaches to the prevention of illnesses and accidents.

The *crime rate* and number of juvenile court cases in a community affect, principally, the mental health of the population; but they also affect the physical health of the population.

An interesting report that demonstrates the value of demographic data to health program planning was prepared by the National Institute of Mental Health (NIMH).[1] Community mental health programs emphasize the provision of diagnostic, treatment, and rehabilitation services at the local level in order to protect the patient's links with family and community and in order to maintain him in his own home and community. Inherent in the success of such a program are certain underlying assumptions: that the patient has a home; that the patient has a family or other persons who are willing, well enough, and financially able to accept responsibility for him and to provide him with the necessary care; that patterns of organization and interpersonal

---

[1] Kramer, Morton. *Applications of Mental Health Statistics.* Geneva, World Health Organization, 1969.

relations in the patient's household will not impede or prevent his recovery and rehabilitation; that the family has sufficient understanding of the patient's illness; that the patient's behavior and needs are such that his presence will not produce undue hardships for others in the household; and that appropriate health and related services are readily accessible to meet the changing needs of patient and family. Thus, data on family characteristics—such as size and composition, employment status of the head and other members of the family, number and age of children living at home, and presence or absence of a spouse or of one or both parents—bear a significant relationship to the rate at which persons of different ages may require psychiatric care. For example, a study[2] in Maryland in the 1960's analyzed rates of first admission to psychiatric facilities for persons living with families by relationship of patient to head of household and number of persons in the home. The data produced by this study indicated that first admission rates were higher for heads of large-sized families; higher for female heads of families; higher for wives of the heads of large families than for wives of heads of small families; higher for children in two-persons families, that is, where at least one parent is absent; and higher for other relatives of the head of family (particularly in two- and three-person families).

These kinds of data about family structure also are needed to estimate the extent of social problems created by mental illness in families and, in addition, to plan for community mental health services. There is a distinct correlation between family structure and length of stay in mental hospitals, which makes it essential to know the expected composition of households to which patients return upon release from the mental hospital, in order to plan follow-up services and to evaluate community placement programs.

ECOLOGIC CHARACTERISTICS

Characteristics of a community's environment that can affect its health are housing and living conditions, water supply and waste disposal services, transportation and travel times, land usage for purposes other than dwellings, zoning, urban renewal plans, topography, and governmental structure—

[2] Klee, Gerald D.; Spiro, Evelyn; Bahn, Anita K.; and Gorwitz, Kurt. "An Ecological Analysis of Diagnosed Mental Illness in Baltimore." Paper presented at the American Psychiatric Association Regional Research Conference on Psychiatric Epidemiology and Mental Health Planning, Baltimore, Md., April 21, 1966.

especially the political decision-making processes. All of these characteristics influence the planning process and the implementation of plans.

Before describing the third characteristic with which health planners are most concerned, namely, the health status of the community, two areas of demographic and ecologic data—their uses and their sources—will be reviewed jointly.

USE OF DEMOGRAPHIC AND ECOLOGIC DATA

The accuracy and, therefore, the usefulness of population projections depend upon the difficult task of assessing future fertility of the population. The United States has relatively low death rates, which will probably continue to decline slowly, although not in sufficient magnitude to appreciably affect population growth in the near future. Fertility levels will thus be the main factor affecting population size.

To a large extent, health needs are age related. Developed nations such as the United States have a higher proportion of older age groups due to declining birth rates as well as to declining death rates among the older population. Also, reductions in infant and childhood mortality have increased the size of the younger age groups.

The population growth rate and its age structure have profound implications on health planning. Newly developing countries have demographic, social, and economic characteristics which limit the choices they can make in planning. Typically, they are struggling to meet service needs of rapidly growing young populations. The greater resources of the developed nations, however, can provide for a wider range of health services to all segments of the population, including older persons with chronic diseases.[3] Nevertheless, it is interesting to note that, within the United States—one of the most highly developed countries in the world—there are communities that have many of the demographic characteristics of newly developing nations: inner city ghettos, isolated rural poverty areas, and Indian reservations.

SOURCES OF DEMOGRAPHIC AND ECOLOGIC DATA

Data relating to demography and ecology derive from two principal types of sources: existing record systems and a canvass of the population.

---

[3] Bright, Margaret. "The Demographic Base for Health Planning." In: Reinke, W. A. *Health Planning: Qualitative Aspects and Quantitative Techniques.* Baltimore, Waverly Press, Inc., 1972. pp. 138–144.

Existing record systems: These systems, which may be tapped for data, are the vital registration system and various administrative record systems from both governmental and private agencies.

1. The *vital registration system* of the United States provides for the collection and legal recording of all births, deaths, marriages, and divorces. It is one of the youngest of such systems among the highly developed nations and has been fully implemented only as recently as 1933, when the last state was admitted to the registration system for births and deaths. Several states still do not report marriages and divorces. About one-half of the world's population lives in communities where registration of births and deaths either is not carried out or is incomplete and, therefore, unreliable for data purposes.

There is a single source of data on vital statistics for all countries—the *Demographic Yearbook of the United Nations*[4]—which classifies the reliability of these data from the various countries, provides information on their completeness and condition of reliability, and, through footnotes, explains the definitions used for easier comparability.

Another system used by some nations is the continuous population register, which is an important source of demographic information. It can provide information that might be considered equivalent to data obtained from a census or a registration of vital statistics. Population registers are not used in the United States.[5]

2. *Administrative record systems* of national and local governmental agencies and private organizations also are good sources of demographic and ecologic data. There are many examples of such record systems, several of which are described here.

An analysis of school enrollments, new electric meter connections, voter registration lists, new dwelling units, etc., will provide statistics on population growth and change in a community. Another governmental record system covers land use data. This usually is available from urban planning offices and includes the following source material:

a. Reference maps, which show streets and other rights-of-way, topog-

4 United Nations Statistical Office. *Demographic Yearbook of the United Nations.* New York, United Nations Publishing Service, 1971.
5 Bright, Margaret. "The Demographic Base for Health Planning." In: Reinke, W. A. *Health Planning: Qualitative Aspects and Quantitative Techniques.* Baltimore, Waverly Press, Inc., 1972. pp. 144–148.

raphy, distribution of property by different types, and similar information.

b. Land use surveys, which can be classified generally as residential (low, medium, high density), retail business, industrial wholesale business, public buildings and open spaces, institutional buildings, and vacant or nonurban use.

c. Vacant land studies, which analyze use capabilities of vacant land, categorized on the basis of topographic features that permit or deter construction of industrial or residential facilities and on the availability of such improvement characteristics as water, sewage, power, highways, etc.

d. Structural and environmental quality surveys, which use an appraisal technique that covers both dwellings and environmental conditions, with a score based on an independent rating of the dwelling for deterioration, safety and sanitation factors, adequacy of heat and light, degree of crowding, etc.; also on a rating of the environment according to land crowding, adequacy of water and sewage services, adequacy of schools and other community facilities, hazards and nuisances, and similar information.

e. Cost revenue studies, which give an indication of how much it would cost to provide public services at various levels of use, as well as revenues that might be realized at various levels of land use, thus giving an indication of the probable fiscal impact of development or redevelopment.

f. Land value studies, which are based on samples of market values and tax assessments and are used to estimate the feasibility of various types of development or redevelopment.

A record system on transportation data also is very important in estimating utilization, along with land use data to determine site locations. Transportation is a major determinant of a population's accessibility to health services. A transportation study might show availability of, and routes for, different modes of transportation.[6]

Other comprehensive types of governmental record systems are those dealing with individuals covered by various social security programs (including Medicare and Medicaid), military inductees and military rejectees, and institutionalized or imprisoned populations.

6 Chapin, F. Stuart, Jr. *Urban Land Use Planning.* Chicago, University of Illinois Press, 1965. Chapter VII.

Population canvass: This second and very important source of demo-graphic and ecologic data is a canvass of the population, which can be accomplished by either a census or a sample survey. The population census is the older method, which generally connotes a total count, whereas the sample survey is a more recent adaptation utilizing sampling theory.

The periodic census, which the United States has been using since 1790, is carried out every 10 years; therefore, it is called the Decennial Census. Sampling was first employed for the 1940 U.S. Census. In the last two Decennial Censuses, a total population count was made for only five items—age, sex, race, relationship to head of household, and marital status—and the remaining data were obtained on a sampling basis. The advantages of a sampling technique are obvious: economy, timeliness (it can be done more frequently since it is on a smaller scale), and quality.

The Decennial Census, conducted by the Census Bureau of the U.S. Department of Commerce, is an enumeration of population and housing and, in past decades, was conducted by direct count. The last Census, in 1970, was conducted largely by mail, a trial run having shown that this method was effective and somewhat cheaper. Special groups, however, can still be handled by enumeration, such as in rural areas where there is a mailing problem or wherever there is a concentration of non-English-speaking or functionally illiterate groups.

Census data in published form are available to some extent in more than 1,000 libraries throughout the country; of these, 137 are designated as census depository libraries. By using these libraries, the cost of purchasing census tapes may be avoided. In contrast to the 1960 Census, the 1970 Census will result in fewer published reports, but there are more data available on computer tapes, and they are available more quickly if one knows how to use a computer or has access to a computer consultant. Summary tapes will cost about $70 per reel, and special tabulations can be purchased for the cost of programming. It is estimated that the average cost of a special tabulation will be about $10,000 (ranging from $500 to $100,000). Census data are available for all sizes of areas, from regions of the country to city blocks and even for block faces—a new grouping in the 1970 Census. Following are the fourteen areas for which data are available:

1. *Regions of the United States:* The northeast region includes the New England and Mid-Atlantic states. The north central region includes the eastern and western north central states. The southern region includes the

South Atlantic and east-south and west-south central states. The western region includes the mountain and Pacific states.

2. *States of the Union.*

3. The *Standard Metropolitan Statistical Area* (SMSA): The SMSA can comprise one city of 50,000 or more and those adjacent counties that are socially and economically integrated with it; it can cross state lines; and it reflects economic and social integration based on where people work, with the adjacent counties often having very sparsely populated areas.

4. *Counties and independent cities.*

5. *Minor Civil Divisions* (MCD); *Census County Divisions* (CCD): These are towns, townships, and arbitrary equivalents.

6. *Congressional districts within the states.*

7. *State Economic Areas* (SEA): There are 509 such areas in the United States.

8. *Economic subregions:* These are combinations of State Economic Areas.

9. *Places*, including cities.

10. *Urbanized areas:* These exclude rural parts of Standard Metropolitan Statistical Areas.

11. *Wards:* Portions of cities, politically oriented.

12. *Census tracts:* Areas with permanent boundaries established by local communities, comprising a homogeneous population of about 4,000 persons per census tract. The census tract often is used in local government data collection programs as well as in the U.S. Census.

13. *City blocks:* Usually, a rectangular piece of land bounded by streets.

14. *Block faces:* A new category in the 1970 Census, it is considered to be one side of a city block.

Table 1, 1970 Population and Housing Census, shows the types of tape files available (counts 1 to 6), the percent coverage of the population and housing, the area covered, the approximate number of such areas in the United States, the approximate number of data items included in each count, and file subdivisions.

The Census is supplemented between decades by the current population survey, which is a monthly sample of 50,000 households in the United States representing $\frac{1}{10}$ of 1 percent of the total population. The current population survey is used to estimate the total population.

In this connection, it should be emphasized that specific small-area data

TABLE 1: 1970 POPULATION AND HOUSING CENSUS, SUMMARY COMPUTER TAPE FILES*

Name of File	Percent of Coverage	Smallest Geographic Area			Approximate No. of Data Items	File Subdivisions
		In File	Average Population Size	Approximate No. in U.S.		
1st Count...	100%	Blockgroup/ED	820	250,000 ED's and Blockgroups	400	File A: BG or ED Summaries File B: State, County, MCD(CCD), MCD-Place, Congressional District
2nd Count...	100%	Tract/MCD(CCD)	Tract: 4,000 MCD's: 200— to 1,000,000+	Tracts 34,600, MCD's (CCD's) 35,000	3,500	File A: Tract Summaries File B: State, County, MCD(CCD), Places, SMSA, and Component Areas
3rd Count...	100%	Block	90	1,500,000	250	Not applicable
4th Count...	15% 5%	Tract/MCD(CCD)	Tract: 4,000 MCD's: 200— to 1,000,000+	Tracts 34,600, MCD's (CCD's) 35,000	13,000 (File A and B, and Places) 30,000 File C (except Places)	File A: Tract Summaries File B: MCD(CCD) Summaries File C: State, County, Places, SMSA, and Component Areas
5th Count...	15% 5%	3- or 5- digit ZIP area	260,000 (3-digit areas), 10,000 (5-digit areas in SMSA's)	788 (3-digit areas), 12,500** (5-digit areas in SMSA's)	800	File A: 3-digit ZIP area File B: 5-digit ZIP areas in SMSA's
6th Count...	15% 5%	Pop. Cities of 100,000+ Hous.—Cities of 50,000+	500,000	132(100,000+) 333(50,000+)	Pop. 150,000 Hous. 110,000	Pop.–Metr. Counties, Non-Metr. Counties 50,000+, Cities 100,000+, Central Cities, SMSA's. Hous.–State, Metr. Counties, Non-Metr. Counties 50,000—, Cities 50,000+, Central Cities, SMSA's.

* Data will be tabulated for the population in 5-digit areas that fall within SMSA's. There is a total of 39,000, 5-digit areas in the United States.
** Adopted from: Gura, Benjamin. "Census Tape Delivery: Dates, Costs, Contents." Paper presented at the Eighth Annual Conference of the Urban and Regional Information Systems Association, September 3–5, 1970, Louisville, Kentucky.

are needed for effective health planning. A sample of national or large-area data is generally much easier to acquire than specific small-area data, but its value is severely limited because of its generalized nature; therefore, it might not be comparable.

Certain demographic data are available as research sources. Listed here are those sources produced as a direct result of census tabulations, as well as those not supplied by census figures.

1. Census products related to demographic data include:

a. *Census of Population Series.* Includes such items as number of inhabitants, population characteristics, social and economic characteristics, detailed characteristics (cross-tabulations), and others of a similar nature.

b. *Subject Reports Series.* Includes data on such special topics as race and child-spacing.

c. *Supplementary Reports Series.* Includes data on such subjects as geographic mobility, poverty areas, and children born.

d. *Monograph Series.* Includes a detailed analysis of such topics as the changing characteristics of the Negro population.

e. *Current Population Reports.* A report of population characteristics by households and families by type; also, population estimates.

f. *Statistical Abstract of the United States.*

g. *County and City Data Book.* Supplements the statistical abstracts.

h. *Census Tracts Series.* Gives population and housing information for small areas within cities (covers 180 cities, most of which have 50,000 or more people).[7,8,9]

2. Other sources of demographic and related data, which are not supplied by the U.S. Census, include:

a. *The Municipal Yearbook,*[10] published by International City Man-

---

[7] U.S. Department of Commerce, Bureau of the Census. *1970 Census Users' Guide.* Washington, D.C., U.S. Government Printing Office, 1970.

[8] U.S. Department of Commerce, Bureau of the Census. *Small-Area Data Notes.* Washington, D.C., U.S. Government Printing Office. Issued periodically.

[9] Gura, Benjamin. "Census Tape Delivery: Dates, Costs, Contents." Paper presented at the Eighth Annual Conference of the Urban and Regional Information Systems Association, September 3–5, 1970, Louisville, Kentucky.

[10] International City Managers Association. *The Municipal Yearbook.* Washington, D.C., 1934– . Annual.

agers Association. Gives independent population estimates and is especially good for small cities.

b. The S. W. Dodge Division of McGraw-Hill Publishing Company, R. L. Polk and Company, and other similar publishing houses. Will sell data on socioeconomic characteristics of selected metropolitan areas. They are basically marketing research firms.

c. Local agencies. Can provide, as previously indicated, data from school districts, utilities, Chambers of Commerce, trade associations, and local governmental agencies; such data will include information from health department registries, newspaper publishing firms, and other local media. The quality and quantity of these data, of course, will vary.

HEALTH STATUS OF A COMMUNITY

Perhaps of greatest importance to the health planner are data which concern those characteristics that relate to the health status of the community. Therefore, the available data on population health will be discussed next. There are two areas to be considered.

The first covers information that is descriptive of the health status of a community and its population. These data are used to assess the unserved needs of the community; to project patterns in changes of use; to establish service priorities; and to analyze causality or, at least, association. They are described briefly as follows:

1. The assessment of unserved needs will depend upon the extent to which diseases, defects, and other health problems are identified and reported.
2. Referring to utilization patterns, an example of data in this area would be the effect that the declining prevalence of tuberculosis has upon the average length of hospital stay, admission rates, occupancy rates, and, ultimately, bed needs.
3. Concerning service priorities, information will include the number of live births, infant death rates, etc., that are used to set priorities for maternal and child health projects.
4. The analysis of causality or, at least, association of factors with disease processes requires cross-tabulations of many characteristics. An example of such data would be the association between an air pollution index and

mortality, morbidity, or disability. Such an example would require the ability to relate demographic, ecologic, and health status data.

The second area covers a number of different types and sources of available data that can be used to describe the health status of population groups. An interesting grouping of these kinds of data follows.

1. *Measurements with a positive tendency.* Include birth and fertility rates and life expectancy.
2. *Measurements with a negative tendency.* Include mortality, morbidity, disability, and some utilization data.

> a. Mortality, in general, is described by crude or overall death rates, or death rates adjusted for age and sex, such as infant and maternal mortality. Mortality also can be described by specific disease rates, that is, the death rates for specific diagnoses. Another measure of death is the proportional mortality ratio, which is the proportion of all deaths due to certain diseases. It is known, for example, that heart diseases, stroke, and cancer comprise 70 percent of all deaths in the United States.
>
> As a general rule, infant mortality is considered a very useful indicator of a population's health level, since, in effect, it is a measure of society's investment in human resources. Because infant mortality is responsive to a multitude of conditions, it is difficult to isolate specific factors influencing a given mortality rate. The major causes of infant deaths include postnatal asphyxia, immaturity and prematurity, congenital malformations, and birth injuries; however, there are many possible control measures that could be used to prevent infant deaths.
>
> Infant mortality rates vary widely throughout the nation and throughout the world, and an increasing number of countries have lower rates than those recorded for the United States. Interpretation of these data requires an understanding of the circumstances of their origin. There are serious limitations to comparing rates, such as nonuniform definitions of birth and infant deaths, variations in promptness of registering live births, and under-registration of births and deaths.[11]
>
> b. Morbidity data measures the incidence and prevalence of disease and other conditions. Incidence of disease is the number of new cases

11 Spiegelman, Mortimer. *Introduction to Demography.* Cambridge, Mass., Harvard University Press, 1970.

occurring during a specified period (usually one year) in a given population. Prevalence of disease is the number of cases that exist in a given population at a single point in time (usually one day, such as the first day of the fiscal year).

Some conditions—particularly certain communicable diseases, certain congenital defects, and birth injuries—are reportable by law to the official health agency for tabulation on a local, state, and national basis. Hospital admissions, health insurance and disability insurance claims, and use of prepaid services—all of which are indicators of utilization of facilities and services—show the types of conditions being experienced by the population. Special surveys of morbidity are used to collect information from the population; these may be via questionnaires or by examination for prevalent disease conditions. Records of absenteeism from school and employment indicate the morbidity level. Special disease registries, such as those for crippled children or for cancer patients, are maintained in connection with specific programs that provide services and follow-up for these patients or for research. A case registry is a central file, sometimes automated, of all cases of a disease or defect, which readily indicates—by some combination of filing and tickler systems—the location of the patient or carrier, the stage of his condition, the date of the next indicated follow-up, and other useful information.

c. Disability data carry morbidity data one step further in relating disease to its effects upon the population. Disabilities include such things as inability to walk, and are generally described in terms of the level of ability to carry on daily activities.

3. *Lack of social well-being, or social pathology.*[12] Evidenced by failure of social or personal adjustment and failure of community organizations. Data with reference to divorce, desertion, alcoholism, drug abuse, crime and delinquency, illegitimacy, prostitution, mental illness, and behavioral and character disorders give some indication of the problems that individuals face in their social or personal adjustments to environment and life circumstances. Unemployment, poverty and deprivation, illiteracy, lack of community resources and services—such as public health, housing, transportation, education, and many others—are evidences of social pathology.

[12] Rogers, Edward. *Human Ecology and Health: An Introduction for Administrators.* 1st Edition. New York, The MacMillan Co., 1960. pp. 103–152, 160–163.

This completes the description of community characteristics relevant to the health status of a community; however, as in the review of data sources covering demographic and ecologic characteristics, the following is a report on sources of health data as an adjunct for continuing study.

SOURCES OF HEALTH STATUS DATA

Sources of health data can be national or local. National data are of little use for local planning except as a point of comparison when used as bases for the evaluation of local conditions.

Data at the National Level: Health statistics from the U.S. National Health Survey (based upon the provisions of the National Health Survey Act, P.L. 84–652, 1956) are a continuing source of health data at the national level. The National Health Survey is performed through weekly interviews with a highly stratified sample of households, using a different sample each week. The weekly samples can be combined to obtain estimates for longer periods of time, for example, one year. Sometimes both questionnaires and interviews are used, and, on occasion, physical examinations also are used for data-collection purposes.

Data from the National Health Survey are published in a series of reports (known as Series 10 to 12 of the *Vital and Health Statistics Reports*, Public Health Service Publication No. 1000).[13] Series 10 includes statistics on illnesses, accidental injuries, and disabilities; use of hospital, medical, dental, and other services; also, other health-related topics, based on data collected in the continuing national Health Interview Survey. Series 11 reports on data from the Health Examination Survey, based on the direct examination, testing, and measurement of national samples of the population. These include the medically defined prevalence of specific diseases and distributions of the population with respect to various physical and physiological measurements. Series 12 reports on data from the Health Records Survey relating to the health characteristics of persons in institutions and on the kind of hospital, medical, nursing, and personal care these persons had received. These findings are based on national samples of establishments providing the afore-

[13] U.S. Department of Health, Education, and Welfare, HSMHA, National Center for Health Statistics. *Vital and Health Statistics Reports.* Series 10 to 12, National Health Survey; Series 11, Health Examination Survey; Series 12, Health Records Survey. Washington, D.C., U.S. Government Printing Office. Published intermittently whenever surveys are completed. Public Health Service Publication No. 1000.

mentioned services and on samples of the resident patients or records of the establishments that were involved in the survey.

Data from the *Report of the National Vital Statistics System*[14] are reported in Series 20 to 23. Series 20 is comprised of various reports on mortality; tabulations by causes of death, age, etc.; and data for geographic areas, states and cities, etc. Series 21 provides data on natality, such as birth by age of mother and birth order. It is compiled by geographic areas, states and cities, etc. Series 22 provides data on marriages and divorces by various demographic factors, geographic areas, etc. Series 23 provides data obtained from the program of sample surveys, related to vital records. The subjects covered in these sample surveys are varied and include such topics as mortality by socioeconomic classes, hospitalization in the last year of life, and X-ray exposure during pregnancy.

A *Monthly Vital Statistics Report*[15] is published by the National Center for Health Statistics of DHEW.

Morbidity and Mortality Weekly Reports[16] are available from the DHEW Center for Disease Control. This resource is located in Atlanta, Georgia, and reports on communicable diseases.

The DHEW *Social Security Bulletin*[17] gives some national data on health expenditures. Similar data can be obtained from records and/or publications of the Blue-Cross/Blue-Shield Plans and/or insurance companies. Such data, for example, appear in the *Source Book of Health Insurance Data*,[18] which is an annual publication of the insurance industry.

The Bureau of Labor Statistics publication, *Consumer Price Index*,[19] gives data on the costs of certain health services.

Data from Local Sources: There are many local sources of health information; among them are the vital statistics registries and registries for certain

14 U.S. Department of Health, Education, and Welfare, HSMHA, National Center for Health Statistics. *Report of the National Vital Statistics System.* Series 20 to 23. Washington, D.C., U.S. Government Printing Office. Published periodically.
15 U.S. Department of Health, Education, and Welfare, HSMHA, National Center for Health Statistics. *Monthly Vital Statistics Report.* Washington, D.C., U.S. Government Printing Office. Monthly.
16 U.S. Department of Health, Education, and Welfare, HSMHA, Center for Disease Control. *Morbidity and Mortality Weekly Report.* Washington, D.C., U.S. Government Printing Office. Weekly.
17 U.S. Department of Health, Education, and Welfare, SSA, Office of Research and Statistics. *Social Security Bulletin.* Washington, D.C., U.S. Government Printing Office, 1938– . Monthly.
18 Health Insurance Institute. *Source Book of Health Insurance Data.* New York, 1972–1973. Annual.
19 U.S. Department of Labor, Bureau of Labor Statistics. *Consumer Price Index.* Washington, D.C., U.S. Government Printing Office, 1913– . Monthly.

diseases such as cancer, venereal diseases, tuberculosis, rheumatic fever, etc. These data usually are available at county, city, and state levels.

Frequently available locally would be data from the Professional Activities Study and Medical Audit Program (PAS-MAP) of the Commission on Professional and Hospital Activities (CPHA).[20] CPHA membership is from the American College of Surgeons, the American College of Physicians, the American Hospital Association, and the Southwestern Michigan Hospital Council, and it is supported by the Kellogg Foundation and by participating hospitals. Through reporting of case abstracts to a central point for tabulation, the CPHA data may be used for evaluation of hospital experience, for evaluation of the quality of medical care, and for determining steps which may be taken to improve the quality of care. The data allow for comparison with other physicians, other departments, and other hospitals.

Another good way to get local data is to conduct a survey. Techniques for collecting general neighborhood data include the windshield survey, consultation with existing community organizations, interviews with representative citizens, and the sample survey.

The *windshield survey* provides a crude estimate of the health situation in a neighborhood by means of observation during a ride or walk through the area. This is an especially useful technique in the summer, when people are outside. One can determine whether the current situation is comparable to that suggested by historical data and can further determine the significant areas needing additional research.

Conversations with neighborhood newspapers, ethnic associations, PTA's, settlement houses, political parties, churches, etc., provide an insight into subjectively felt problems, needs, desires, and recommendations. Although such groups and organizations generally are very familiar with the community, it must be remembered that they may have a biased point of view.

Interviews with representative residents, merchants, bartenders, barbers, policemen, etc., also provide useful information; however, it is frequently found that people have been "surveyed to death" and do not like to have their hopes raised needlessly.

Sample surveys give a truly representative picture of what is happening in the community. They are expensive and time-consuming, but a small sample can be made very accurately by careful design and implementation. A com-

[20] Commission on Professional and Hospital Activities. Professional Activities Study and Medical Audit Program. Ann Arbor, Michigan.

munity sample survey has three phases: organizing the survey group, conducting the survey itself, and data analysis.

1. *Organizing the survey group.* This group should be comprised of persons with technical competence, consumers, and members of agencies with access to relevant data. A steering committee and technical subcommittees are useful for planning a broad-based survey, in addition to a technical staff to handle the survey techniques, data analysis, and report writing.

2. *Conducting the survey.* The area to be covered must be precisely defined, and the types of information to be gathered must be decided in advance. There are many guides available for this purpose. It is important, before starting, to identify gaps in available information. The appropriate survey technique should be selected: it may be a mailed questionnaire, a telephone interview, or a personal interview.

The mailed questionnaire usually has a low response rate because of disinterest, functional illiteracy, or other reasons; however, it is relatively inexpensive. It generally is preferable for organizational respondents rather than for individual respondents. The telephone survey overcomes some of the low-response problems of the mailed questionnaire, but not everyone has a telephone, and many persons are suspicious of an unknown interviewer.

The personal interview is more expensive because of manpower costs; it is also slower and takes longer to complete. The interviewers require thorough training and close supervision, including spot-checking through a reinterview by another person. Interviews should be similar to the interviewees in racial, ethnic, and class characteristics in order to maximize the response.

The interviewees or the population to be sampled should be selected on a random basis; the sample can be a cluster or stratified sample. Any sample type must be based on a random process in order to permit valid statistical analyses of the results. The size of the probability sample affects the interpretation of the results.

3. *Data analysis.* It is very important that the data collection instrument or questionnaire be prepared in advance. It can contain open-ended or closed questions. The length must be carefully evaluated to ensure both maximum information and maximum response. Some questions may be used for cross-checking—for example, those on income and occupation—and should yield compatible answers. The data collection instrument must

be pretested and revised, if necessary, before it is used for the main survey.

It is helpful to design the questionnaire for easy coding, or even precoding, in order to simplify the data analysis. The analyst must have a good understanding of the subject matter so he will not make profound errors, for example, confusing association with causality.

A sophisticated example of the community survey process is the Neighborhood Environmental Evaluation and Decision System (NEEDS). The NEEDS program is based on the concept that a health problem usually arises from a combination of different factors. NEEDS is an excellent method for statistically relating numerous variables of personal and family health to environmental factors and elements. A three-phase community survey gathers data on neighborhood quality, housing quality, and household health in a stratified, two-stage cluster sample. The forms, training, and processing for such a study may be furnished by the U.S. Public Health Service, but data collection is done by the community. NEEDS can be repeated as often as necessary, for benchmarks in the evaluation process, for points-in-time in longitudinal studies, and for assessing changes in the community between the Decennial Censuses.[21]

INTERRELATIONSHIPS AND LINKAGES OF DATA

A problem arises in the use of demographic, ecologic, and health status data for a specific locale when establishing linkages of the several types of data for specific geographic locations with one another.

A useful tool is *A Geographic Base File for Urban Data Systems,*[22] which describes the geography of an area (streets, intersections, geographic codes, addresses) in computer-readable form. The *File* is designed to relate facts to their geographic location and is constructed to produce printouts of data in the form of computer mappings. There are four types of mappings: the grid system approach, based on the latitude-longitude concept of map making; the parcel/block inventory system, using established physical and legal

---

[21] U.S. Department of Health, Education, and Welfare, PHS, Bureau of Community Environment Management. *"NEEDS," Neighborhood Environmental Evaluation and Decision System.* Washington, D.C., U.S. Government Printing Office, 1971.

[22] System Development Corporation. *A Geographic Base File for Urban Data Systems.* Santa Monica, Calif., 1969. Based upon a slide presentation by Robert Totschek, V. Almendinger, and K. Needham at May 21, 1969 meeting of BAAISCC (Bay Area Automated Information System Coordinating Committee).

boundaries; the Address Coding Guide (ACG),[23] relating coded information on the residential address to block face or block or census tract; and the Dual Independent Map Encoding (DIME)[24] approach, combining the address information from the ACG files with information describing the urban street network. The ACG is not suitable for computer mapping because it does not include coordinated information. The DIME approach, however, ensures that the entire area is covered by the system. The DIME file may be developed in one of two ways: directly from census metropolitan and local address maps or by augmenting ACG information with DIME features.

Since the DIME approach plus ACG information produce the most comprehensive data for a specific locale, this system is discussed here in some detail.

The ACG-DIME file makes possible the interrelationship of urban data by geographic location, allowing for cross-references and cross-correlations of such matters as employment, land parcels, health data, facility inventories, traffic accidents, transport networks, topographic data, survey data, census data, precinct data, school districts, and postal zones. A system of this type can be used in many areas, including transportation, health, and school planning; housing and community analysis; and law enforcement. For example: the mapping of urban data by computer; the association of information on activities or occurrences that can be identified by address with other urban data, for comparative analysis; special census tabulations to aid in specifying areal aggregations of the basic record data for both individuals and housing units; utilization of a control framework for a land use inventory; and, with the addition of travel time for each segment of the file, the ACG-DIME system can be used as a model to determine optimal routes for emergency vehicles. The City of New Haven, Connecticut,[25] for example, is using such a system to correlate address data from the Census, the family health survey, vital records, and hospital obstetrical records for the purpose of maternal and child health planning and programming.

The Community Profile Data Center, which is one of the Community Health Services of the Health Services and Mental Health Administration

---

23 Files prepared by the Census Bureau and local agencies for use in some metropolitan areas participating by mail in the 1970 Decennial Census.
24 Developed and utilized in the New Haven, Connecticut, Census Use Study.
25 U.S. Department of Commerce, Bureau of the Census. *Census Use Study: Family Health Survey, Report No. 6,* 1969; *Health Information System, Report No. 7,* 1969; and *Health Information System II, Report No. 12,* 1971. Washington, D.C., U.S. Government Printing Office.

(HSMHA), will prepare, upon request, community profiles for defined geographic areas, utilizing the health resources inventory data as its research base. The Community Profile Data Center does not function as a primary data collection organization; rather, it attempts to rely on the acquisition and use of data collected by other groups. The Center prepares small-area data analyses for counties and smaller areas.

COMMUNITY RESOURCES

A community's resources basically are of three types—men, money, and materials. The productivity of each of these resources is as important as the quantity that is available. For example, manpower productivity may be expanded by the assignment of new duties to existing manpower, by the development of new types of health manpower, and by the redistribution of manpower resources. The productivity of facilities also may be expanded by new techniques, systems, procedures, equipment, types, and locations; for example, better matching of patients with facilities and services through an automated patient placement system.

Demand for resources is a derived demand and, therefore, the interest is on productivity and not on the resources per se. An example would be the number of patients that can be cared for by a specific physician per year. The number of beds per 1,000 population, however, is not a description of productivity.

Current demand for resources is estimated by such things as:

1. *Counting vacant budgeted positions:* Data on these positions can be misleading unless it is known which positions are relatively impossible to fill because of real manpower shortages.

2. *Checking regional distribution for imbalances:* Using physicians as an example, their types of specialities as well as their types of practices and sources of patients served must be taken into consideration to satisfy regional imbalances.

3. *Checking program services for imbalances:* Data on such services can be misleading unless the resources are pinpointed geographically, with due consideration given to the size, capacity, and population base of a facility. An example of program imbalance would be heavy emphasis on acute hospital care at the expense of adequate home care and ambulatory care.

MANPOWER

Manpower resources are the subject of Chapter 8.

FINANCES

Money as a health resource is derived from either private funds or public sources of health funding. This resource, too, is in limited supply.

1. *Private funds* may come from such sources as direct payments by the user to the provider, indirect payments through pooled funds and risk sharing (insurance) to the provider, philanthropy, and expenditures by industry for services.

2. *Public sources of health funding* may include tax appropriations for direct provision of services, tax appropriations for subsidy payments, tax appropriations for purchase of services, and collection and disbursement of social insurance contributions by public authorities. Public funds for health services are dependent upon the tax base. In urban centers today, where the tax base is insufficient because of poor socioeconomic conditions, funds are becoming even more scarce for essential public services for the citizens of these jurisdictions. Furthermore, urban residents are placed in competition with commuters and visitors who, although they spend much of their time in the urban area and use the available services, reside and pay taxes in the surrounding suburbs.

Virtually all sources of funds derive ultimately from the local community through taxes, charges, or contributions. When making major contributions, the public expects to have a voice in determining how the funds they have contributed shall be allocated.

In measuring financial resources, both capital financing and operating costs must be taken into account. With respect to capital financing, the planner must consider the tax base, current bonded indebtedness, legal limits on taxes and bonds, past success with fund drives, and the possibility of large-scale contributions or endowments. With respect to the availability of resources for meeting operating costs, the planner must consider the annual per capita and per family income; the availability of public or private payments and their volume and adequacy; the volume and coverage of health insurance; the economic stability of the area (anticipated economic fluctuations and unemployment); and the public attitude toward health care (willingness to use and pay for facilities and services).

The once widely held belief that the burden of health care payments should fall upon those who directly benefit has shifted generally toward the concept that each citizen has a right to needed health care. Financing health care through insurance contributions, sales taxes, or property taxes is either inequitable or inadequate; thus, the tendency today is to rely increasingly upon the government for general revenues.

Therefore, to assess the financing capability of a community, it is important to estimate its tax capacity and its economic standing and stability. A good example is a recent analysis of intercounty differences in economic status by the state of Georgia for the purpose of measuring relative financing capability per capita.[26,27] The following procedures were used.

The first step was to examine several economic and demographic variables: the 21 to 64 age groups—that is, the approximate working-age population; the effective buying income; the total adjusted gross income—that is, minus business expense—as shown by Georgia income tax data; total assessed values for general property from Georgia property tax data; and number of persons receiving public assistance payments.

The next step was to compare the percentage of each county's state total for each variable with that of Georgia's population. Indexes were derived from these comparisons, and the counties were ranked according to the computed index numbers. The county group designations (rank) take account of a combined weighted index, as well as checklists showing the county's ranking with respect to each variable. The relative ranking of some counties varied considerably according to different indicators. For these counties, therefore, it was necessary to make additional comparisons between a given county's share of Georgia's 1970 population and that county's share of insured wages and of persons on Medicaid rolls, respectively.

Finally, after ranking, the counties were distributed among seven groups, ranging from the most to the least affluent. To judge how affluent the top-rated counties are, Georgia's statewide average was used as the standard of comparison.

Over the past decade, the Advisory Commission on Intergovernmental Relations,[28] a federally funded agency, has been examining and testing ways

[26] White, E. Lamar. *Provisional Affluence Ratings of Georgia Counties.* Office of Comprehensive Health Planning, Georgia Department of Public Health, December 1971.
[27] Butler, Karen. *A Method for Geographic Analysis of Target Areas.* Office of Comprehensive Health Planning, Georgia Department of Public Health, December 1971.
[28] Advisory Commission on Intergovernmental Relations. *Measuring the Fiscal Capacity and Effort of State and Local Areas.* Washington, D.C., U.S. Government Printing Office, 1971. No. M–58.

to measure the relative financing capability of state governments and the extent to which they actually use this capability. Improved measures of fiscal capacity and fiscal effort led the Commission to recommend—both to the Federal Government and to the states—that they increase emphasis on equalization of local resources in the distribution of their grants among eligible jurisdictions. Also, the Commission has urged state and local governments to make more effective use of their revenue resources and to encourage, in various ways, the mitigation of interstate and interlocal tax load differentials.

Traditionally, two kinds of economic indicators have been used to measure relative fiscal capacity and tax effort: estimates of per capita personal income and estimates of taxable property values on the local area tax rolls. These indicators, although useful, leave much to be desired. At state level, for example, resident personal income fails to reflect closely the potential of certain revenue sources such as severance taxes, motor fuel taxes, and gambling taxes; locally, the property tax base pertains only to a portion of available financing resources; and, nationally, about two-fifths of all own-source revenue of local governments is obtained from nonproperty sources.

The need for meaningful comparative measures of fiscal capacity and effort—that is, their actual or potential value for grant-in-aid use—was a major objective for studies by the Advisory Commission on Intergovernmental Relations. While federal grants made directly to local governments have been multiplying in variety and dollar amount, these federal-local aid arrangements, unlike some important federal-state grant programs, do not provide for any differentiation between jurisdictions of relatively low capacity or high effort. Lacking any organized body of statistics to reflect the relative fiscal capacity of claimant local areas of governments, it has been necessary, in the design of federal-local aid arrangements, to disregard such differences. If, however, meaningful comparative measures of fiscal capacity and effort can be developed for various local areas and jurisdictions, then new policy options might be available for the design and administration of federal-local grants. The Commission has concluded that meaningful and useful comparisons of the relative fiscal capacity and effort of various local areas can be made.

The process of estimating the tax capacity of particular areas involves the following steps:

1. Determine the inclusiveness of the term taxes, and determine which tax classes should be handled separately.

2. Review current state and local practices with regard to each type of tax in order to ascertain its predominant or representative form.

3. Locate tax-base data for each tax or, in the absence of such data, assemble quantitative information about some measure that could reasonably be taken to represent the actual base.

4. Obtain an average rate for each tax by dividing its nationwide yield by the nationwide base or its proxy.

5. Calculate the capacity (potential yield of each tax class for particular areas—states, SMSAs, and counties) by applying the average rate to the base measure for such areas.

6. Add capacity figures thus developed for particular taxes in each area to arrive at the area's total tax capacity. This procedure is described in detail in the March 1971 report on *Measuring the Fiscal Capacity and Effort of State and Local Areas* prepared by the Advisory Commission on Intergovernmental Relations.[29] Also discussed in the report are the procedures for measuring the capacity for nontax revenue sources and for measuring revenue efforts.

FACILITIES

In assessing the availability of facilities, an inventory should be made, to include the total number, type (such as hospital, extended care, or ambulatory facility), size, services offered (some services, such as visiting nurses, are not offered in a facility), staffing, utilization, and admission policies and practices (such as religious or ethnic barriers to utilization).

Also, projections of the supply of, and demand for, the facilities must be made. Projections of the supply of facilities can be made by reviewing the Hill-Burton Plan, which calculates needs and recommends priorities, and by interviews with heads of existing agencies regarding proposed expansion and the possible entrance of competitor facilities into the area. The projection of demand for, or utilization of, the facilities can be based upon anticipated population increases, changes in technology, and styles of practice. For example, the advent and widespread use of antibiotics over the last several decades has changed hospital utilization for treatment of communicable diseases. More recently, the widespread use of birth control measures and, still

---

29 Advisory Commission on Intergovernmental Relations. *Measuring the Fiscal Capacity and Effort of State and Local Areas.* Washington, D.C., U.S. Government Printing Office, 1971. No. M–58.

more recently, the introduction of abortion services have changed the utilization rate for obstetrical beds.

The Hill-Burton Program *Grants Manual*[30] is an excellent and widely used source of uniform procedures for accounting for existing beds (that is, bed capacity) and evaluating existing facilities for modernization. It also describes a method for determining bed needs for inpatient facilities.

The *Public Health Service Regulations* pertaining to the construction and modernization of hospital and medical facilities (that is, the Hill-Burton Regulations)[31] set forth general minimum requirements for construction and equipment. These requirements are necessary to ensure properly planned and well-constructed hospitals and public health centers which can be maintained efficiently and operated to furnish adequate services. All projects for which federal assistance is requested must be in conformance with these regulations or, as commonly stated, must meet the criteria for conforming beds.

FACILITIES CRITERIA FOR FEDERAL ASSISTANCE

The standards required by the Federal Government provide for a site survey and soil investigation, as well as for approval of the site location and specific criteria for each unit of the general hospital and other facilities.

The criteria for assuring general hospital conformance include requirements for the administration department, adjunct diagnostic and treatment facilities (laboratory, radiology, pharmacy, etc.), nursing department (nursing units, treatment rooms, etc.), nursery department, surgical department, obstetrics department, emergency department, service department (dietary facilities, housekeeping, etc.), outpatient department, pediatric nursing unit, psychiatric unit, plus other, more general, requirements. The requirements for each are described in detail according to the size of the facility.

During the course of planning and the actual construction or remodeling, the state agency must make adequate periodic inspections and certify to conformance with the regulations.

---

30 U.S. Department of Health, Education, and Welfare, HSMHA, Health Care Facilities Service. *Health Services Grants Manual, Title II, Construction and Modernization of Hospital and Medical Facilities.* Washington, D.C., U.S. Government Printing Office. Revised periodically according to need.
31 U.S. Department of Health, Education, and Welfare. *Public Health Service Regulations— Part 53.* Washington, D.C., U.S. Government Printing Office, 1965.

UTILIZATION REVIEW

Utilization review is a system for measuring the productivity of hospitals and other health facilities, thereby ultimately measuring their effectiveness. It is required for certification of the facility to participate in Medicare and Medicaid reimbursement under Titles 18 and 19 of the Social Security Act. The utilization review plan focuses on sampling admissions, duration of stay, and professional services furnished by types of cases. By assessing the quality and cost of care, the utilization review process provides continuing medical education as well as improvement in hospital administrative procedures. Hopefully, this should result in better utilization of scarce resources and in stabilizing costs by providing the most appropriate level of care for each patient according to his current need.

SOURCES OF DATA ON FACILITIES

Some sources of data and information about facilities are: the annual *Guide Issue* of the *Journal of the American Hospital Association; Health Resources Statistics*, reported annually by the National Center for Health Statistics of HSMHA/DHEW; the *Directory of Non-Federal Statistics for States and Local Areas;*[32] the Hill-Burton *Grants Manual* and the State Plan of the Hill-Burton Agency, which show conforming and nonconforming bed ratios for hospitals and related facilities; reports based on the Master Facility Inventory Survey of the National Center for Health Statistics;[33] publications of the Community Profile Data Center,[34] as described in the brochure, *Data Available from the Community Profile Data Center;* miscellaneous sources, such as telephone listings, and visits to agencies and associations, such as the Hospital Association and comprehensive health planning agencies.

Several problems arise in attempting to assess the availability of facilities as health resources. The planner will find that frequently, especially with reference to nursing homes and related facilities, definitions are not standardized. Thus, it is difficult to distinguish among extended care facilities, nursing homes, etc., all of which may sound alike but may offer entirely different kinds of services. It is difficult also to judge the quality of a facility

---

[32] U.S. Department of Commerce, Bureau of the Census. *Directory of Non-Federal Statistics for State and Local Areas: 1969.* Washington, D.C., U.S. Government Printing Office, 1970.
[33] U.S. Department of Health, Education, and Welfare, HSMHA, National Center for Health Statistics, Division of Health Resources. Reports based on the Master Facility Inventory Survey. Washington, D.C., U.S. Government Printing Office. Issued periodically.
[34] U.S. Department of Health, Education, and Welfare, HSMHA, Community Health Service. The Community Profile Data Center, Parklawn Building, Rockville, Md. 20852.

since, frequently, there are no set standards, except those of the Hill-Burton program.

The planner will find that some states do not report all facilities to the National Center for Health Statistics through the annual reporting system. In some states, facilities such as homes for the aged and homes for dependent children are not tabulated. States vary in the amount of control they exercise over various types of facilities. Sometimes, instead of one central licensing agency for all health and health-related facilities, control may be divided among several state agencies; therefore, several different agencies must be approached for information about facilities. Furthermore, these kinds of information are gathered and tabulated at different frequencies and thus might not be equally current.

REFERENCES

1. Berg, Robert L. et al. "Bed Utilization Studies for Community Planning." *Journal of the American Medical Association, 207*(13):2411–2413, March 31, 1969.

2. Carner, Donald C. *Planning for Hospital Expansion and Remodelling.* Springfield, Ill., C. C. Thomas, 1968. pp. 70–85.

3. Cashman, John; Maki, Nancy; and Logsdon, Ruth. "Utilization Review: Whose Responsibility? What Are Its Potentials?" *Hospital Progress,* June 1968, pp. 74–86.

4. Egan, Douglas M. *Physician Productivity, Personnel Utilization and Physician Income.* Denver, Medical Group Management Association, 1969.

5. Friedan, Bernard J. and Peters, James. "Urban Planning and Health Services: Opportunities for Cooperation." American Institute of Planners *AIP Journal, 36*(2):82–94, March 1970.

6. Hamburg, A.Z. "Using Census Data in Local Planning." *Hospitals, 41*: 60–65, September 16, 1967.

7. House of Delegates of the American Hospital Association. "AHA House Approves Financial Statement." *Hospitals, 43*:23–26, March 1, 1969.

8. Kirsch, Arnold I. et al. "New Proxy Measure for Health Status." *Health Services Research, 4*(3):223–230, Fall 1969.

9. McGibony, John R., M.D. *Principles of Hospital Administration.* New York, G.P. Putnam's Sons, 1969. pp. 38–53.

10. Mills, Alden B. *Functional Planning of General Hospitals.* New York, McGraw-Hill, 1969. pp. 43–63.
11. Palmiere, Darwin. "Community-Based Approaches to Utilization Review." *Public Health Reports, 83*(9): 705–707, September 1968.
12. Pressler, Stanley, Everette, and Ray. *Financial Implications for Hospitals in Comprehensive Health Planning.* Bloomington, Indiana University, Bureau of Business Research, 1968. pp. 203–214.
13. Spiegelman, Mortimer. *Introduction to Demography.* Cambridge, Mass., Harvard University Press, 1968. pp. 8–42, 171–221.
14. Tayback, Matthew and Levin, Peter. "Urban Health Crisis: Management of the Public's Health Investment." *American Journal of Public Health, 59*(12):2221–2226, December 1969.
15. U.S. Department of Health, Education, and Welfare. *Health Resources Statistics.* Washington, D.C., 1968. pp. 307, 215–219.
16. Wallace, Helen M. et al. "Availability and Usefulness of Selected Health and Socioeconomic Data for Community Planning." *American Journal of Public Health, 57*(5):762–771, May 1967.
17. Walters, R.F., Ph.D. and Bunch, O.E., M.S. "Utilization of Provisional Discharge Diagnoses to Enhance Patient Traffic-Pattern Studies." *Medical Care, 7*(4):313–326, July–August 1969.
18. Wenkert, Walter. "Communications: Concepts and Methodology in Planning Patient Care Services." *Medical Care, 7*(4):327–331, July–August 1969.

8
CHAPTER

MANPOWER

This chapter on health manpower planning is divided into three sections. The first will delineate the manpower system, the second will deal with problems inherent in projecting manpower needs, and the third will outline a systems approach to the manpower problem.

THE MANPOWER SYSTEM

The problem of providing and maintaining a continually growing and properly distributed supply of health manpower has been for many years a major concern of health policy makers and health planners. Although the health manpower problem is recognized today, there is little solidarity of opinion on what causes the problem. There also is little understanding of the scope of the health manpower system and how it works. Therefore, this chapter will first present some ideas concerning the manpower system.

Health manpower is the most significant part of the cost and operation of today's health system. Manpower accounts for an estimated 65 to 70 percent of hospital costs, 70 to 80 percent of costs in doctors' offices, and 90 percent or more of nursing home costs.[1] With the increasing concern over the cost of medical care, it is not surprising that the health manpower system is of major importance.

Taken in a historical context, health manpower has often been equated with physician manpower. Although the physician has been considered to be the primary health worker and has been the subject of much of the writings on health manpower, he is only a small part of the total health manpower scheme. In 1900, approximately 2 out of 3 health workers were physicians; by 1965, this figure had become 1 out of 10; and by 1970, the figure was 1

---

[1] Hoff, Wilbur. "Resolving the Health Manpower Crisis: A Systems Approach to Utilizing Personnel." *American Journal of Public Health, 61*(12):2491–2504, December 1971.

out of 13. Projections for 1975 estimate a further reduction, possibly to 1 out of 20 or 25. Although the physician ratio in health manpower continues to decrease, other health occupations are increasing. Table 2 gives a partial listing of the occupations included in the health field, divided into 32 major categories.

TABLE 2: PARTIAL LIST OF HEALTH OCCUPATIONS

1. Administration
   Health Administrator
   Health Program Analyst
   Health Systems Analyst
2. Biomedical Engineering
   Biomedical Engineer
   Biomedical Engineering Technician
   Biomedical Engineering Aide
3. Chiropractic and Naturopathy
   Chiropractor
   Naturopath
4. Clinical Laboratory Services
   Clinical Laboratory Scientist
   Clinical Laboratory Technologist
   Clinical Laboratory Technician
   Clinical Laboratory Aide
5. Dentistry and Allied Services
   Dentist
   Dental Hygienist
   Dental Assistant
   Dental Laboratory Technician
6. Dietetic and Nutritional Services
   Dietician
   Nutritionist
   Dietary Technician
   Dietary Aide
   Food Service Supervisor
7. Environmental Health Services
   Environmental Scientist
   Environmental Engineer
   Environmental Technologist
   Environmental Technician
   Environmental Aide
8. Food and Drug Protective Services
   Food Technologist
   Food and Drug Inspector
   Food and Drug Analyst
9. Health Education
   Health Educator
   Health Education Aide

10. Information and Communication
    Health Information Specialist
    Health Science Writer
    Health Technical Writer
    Medical Illustrator
11. Library Services
    Medical Librarian
    Medical Library Assistant
    Hospital Librarian
12. Mathematical Sciences
    Mathematician
    Statistician
13. Medical Record Services
    Medical Record Librarian
    Medical Record Technician
    Medical Record Clerk
14. Medicine and Osteopathy
    Physician
    Osteopathic Physician
15. Midwifery
    Midwife
16. Natural Sciences
    Anatomist
    Botanist
    Chemist
    Ecologist
    Entomologist
    Epidemiologist
    Geneticist
    Hydrologist
    Immunologist
    Meteorologist
    Microbiologist
    Nutritionist
    Oceanographer
    Pathologist
    Pharmacologist
    Physicist
    Physiologist
    Sanitary Sciences Specialist
    Zoologist

17. Nursing and Related Services
    Nurse
    Practical Nurse
    Nursing Aide
    Orderly
    Attendant
    Home Health Aide
    Ward Clerk
18. Occupational Therapy
    Occupational Therapist
    Occupational Therapy Assistant
    Occupational Therapy Aide
19. Orthotic and Prosthetic Technology
    Orthotist
    Orthotic Aide
    Prosthetist
    Prosthetic Aide
    Restoration Technician
20. Pharmacy
    Pharmacist
    Pharmacy Aide
21. Physical Therapy
    Physical Therapist
    Physical Therapy Assistant
    Physical Therapy Aide
22. Podiatry
    Podiatrist
23. Radiologic Technology
    Radiologic Technologist
    Radiologist Technician
24. Secretarial and Office Services
    Secretary
    Office Assistant
25. Social Sciences
    Anthropologist
    Economist
    Psychologist
    Sociologist
26. Social Work
    Clinical Social Worker
    Clinical Social Work Assistant
    Clinical Social Work Aide
27. Specialized Rehabilitation Services
    Corrective Therapist
    Corrective Therapy Aide
    Education Therapist
    Manual Arts Therapist

    Music Therapist
    Recreation Therapist
    Recreation Therapy Aide
    Homemaking Rehabilitation
        Consultant
28. Speech Pathology and Audiology
    Audiologist
    Speech Pathologist
29. Veterinary Medicine
    Veterinarian
    Veterinary Technician
30. Vision Care
    Ophthalmologist
    Optometrist
    Vision Care Technologist
    Orthoptic Technician
    Optician
    Visual Care Aide
31. Vocational Rehabilitation Counseling
    Vocational Rehabilitation
        Counselor
32. Miscellaneous Health Services
    Assistance for Physicians
        Physician's Associate
        Physician's Assistant
        Physician's Aide
    Emergency Health Service
        Medical Emergency Technician
        Ambulance Attendant (Aide)
    Inhalation Therapy
        Inhalation Therapist
        Inhalation Therapy Aide
    Medical Machine Technology
        Cardiopulmonary Technician
        Electrocardiograph Technician
        Electroencephalograph
            Technician
        Other
    Nuclear Medicine
        Nuclear Medical Technologist
        Nuclear Medical Technician
    Other Health Services
        Community Health Aide
        Extracorporeal Circulation
            Specialist
        Other

The bulk of the growth in health manpower during the last decade has been in the allied health occupations.[2] Between 1965 and 1967, the allied health worker pool increased by 26 percent, or by almost 500,000 people, as a result of the greater demand for medical care, the split of existing jobs, the expansion of jobs, and the introduction of new technology in the medical field. It was noted that, in this same period, the supply of doctors, dentists, and registered nurses increased by only 6 percent.[3]

The growth of the allied health field has been seen by some observers as a filling-in of the gap between highly trained physicians and lesser trained health personnel. This filling-in process is needed to free the many doctors and nurses who are wasting their time and skills performing functions that lesser trained allied health personnel can easily handle.

A SCHEMATIC REPRESENTATION OF HEALTH MANPOWER

In the economic sense, health manpower is a resource. Since it is a scarce resource, it should be given close attention in order to ensure optimal resource allocation. In this context, the most important considerations are supply and demand structures and resource utilization factors.

Figure 6 is a schematic representation of the health manpower system. There are three major interacting components of this representation: A – the demand structure, B – the market, and C – the supply structure. The interaction among these factors is indicated in the figure by the arrows. This uncomplicated schematic can be followed step by step.

First, the demand for medical care determines the demand for health manpower. Next, supply and utilization of manpower interact and, taken together, determine the availability of health manpower. Therefore, the surplus or deficit between the demand for manpower and the availability of manpower affects the components, which need to be stimulated to increase or decrease the availability of manpower. Then, because the disparity between supply and demand cannot be measured precisely, it is determined by estimation. Finally, based on the estimation, manpower planning decisions are made, and legislation may be enacted to effect the delivery of care (and, hence, the demand for manpower), the supply and utilization of manpower, and the availability of manpower.

---

[2] "Allied health occupations" is used here to refer to all health occupations other than doctors, dentists, and licensed nurses.
[3] Acton, Jan and Levine, Robert. *State Health Manpower Planning: A Policy Overview.* Santa Monica, Calif., The RAND Corporation, 1971.

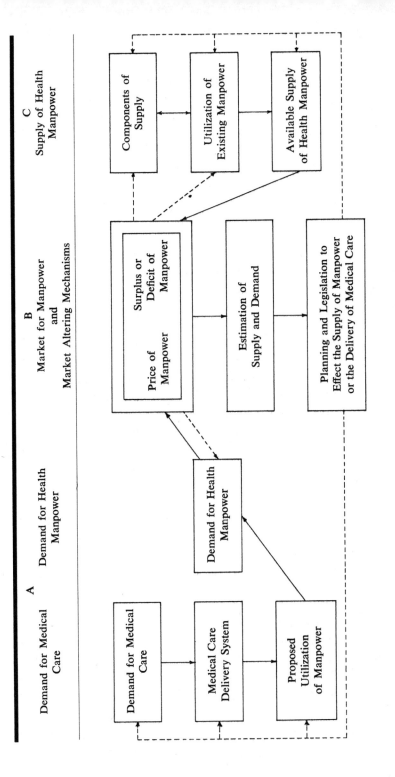

Figure 6: Schematic representation of the health manpower mechanism

Adapted from: Butter, Irene. "Health Manpower Research: A Survey." *Inquiry*, 4(4):5–41, December 1967.

The relative simplicity of the diagram should not suggest that the system itself is simple. Health manpower is a complex system with numerous exogenous variables to complicate the health planner's task. The major components of the diagram will be discussed further.

DEMAND FOR MEDICAL CARE AND HEALTH MANPOWER

The demand for health manpower is a derived demand, which means that there is no demand for such manpower on the part of the consuming public. There is, however, a primary demand for medical care. Medical care is delivered through a delivery system by health manpower. Thus, the demand for manpower is derived from the demand for medical care.

The demand for medical care is very dynamic, complicating the determination of demand for manpower in several ways. There are three sets of factors that can be identified as affecting manpower demand: demand for health care services, the delivery system providing the care, and the proposed utilization of individual health professions.[4] The demand for health care services is, in part, a function of the socioeconomic and demographic characteristics of the population in any area. The delivery system affects demand since different subsystems deliver different levels of care, that is, a doctor's office versus a hospital. Finally, the utilization of a profession affects demand: for example, if all doctors decided to work 20 hours per week and to see only one patient per hour, the number of doctors demanded would shift significantly.

SUPPLY COMPONENTS

There are a number of components that affect the available supply of manpower. This section will expand on some of the more important factors. The first two are closely related: recruitment and training capacity. The first determinant of supply in any occupation is the number of persons willing to enter that occupation. Once a number of persons have been recruited, they must be trained. There are limited training facilities, however, which may restrict entry to the occupation. The present physician situation is classic in this sense. There are many persons willing to enter the field, but training capacity is limited in U.S. medical schools.

Licensure, another supply component, effectively blocks entry into the medical profession. There are basically two sides to this argument: the pro-

---

[4] Butter, Irene. "Health Manpower Research: A Survey." *Inquiry*, 4(4):5–41, December 1967.

tective and the restrictive. Licensure may be necessary to protect the consumer and, thus, is needed. There is much room, however, to dispute who should control the licensure procedure. If it is to protect the consumer, should not the consumer help control licensure, rather than the professional societies alone? In the past, licensure has probably been more restrictive for nurses and dentists than for physicians. Medical school enrollments have been the major restrictive force in controlling entry into the medical profession.[5]

To avoid a long discourse on economics and social factors related to the supply of health manpower, it should be sufficient to state that these factors affect supply. Remuneration, occupational goals, and the retention rate within an occupation category—all have a short- and long-range effect on supply. Some long-range considerations that may not be immediately visible are the cost of a medical education, the length of the educational experience, the probability of completing training once it is started, and the projected future earnings of the occupation.[6]

The final aspect of supply worthy of mention is international migration. The United States is attracting a substantial number of foreign-trained doctors and other health professionals. In 1970, it was estimated that about 30 percent of the doctors in approved internships and residencies were graduates of foreign medical schools (this includes U.S. citizens educated in foreign schools). In 1969, 23 percent of the almost 10,000 newly licensed doctors were educated in foreign schools. This influx can be considered a subsidy to the U.S. manpower pool, in that it provides manpower whose training costs were paid for in another country. It has, however, alienated some foreign medical communities that have lost doctors through migration.

UTILIZATION

The utilization of available manpower is a topic receiving increased attention. A number of studies are attempting to determine how the productivity of health manpower can be increased. One of the major discussions concerning manpower utilization centers on the MEDEX program for returning military medical corpsmen. This program attempts to increase the productivity of existing physicians through the use of medical corpsmen as physician assistants. It has been proven that a number of the functions performed by the highly trained physician can be performed just as easily by assistants who

[5] Butter, Irene. "Health Manpower Research: A Survey." *Inquiry,* *4*(4):5–41, December 1967.
[6] *Ibid.*

have had less training. Thus, the physician is able to devote more of his time to problems that require his level of competence. By 1971, the MEDEX program had placed more than 1,900 medical corpsmen as physician assistants.

The utilization of complementary and substitute manpower is not limited to the physician field. It has been observed in the nursing profession over a number of years and is also evident in a number of other health occupations. It has been suggested that nursing care in hospitals has shifted downward by a full level. The job formerly performed by a registered nurse is now done by a practical nurse, and the practical nurse's job has been taken over by a nurse's aide.

Other factors that relate to utilization are institutional in nature. The size of the organization and the organizational configuration that will allow optimal utilization of the health staff have been subjects of much study by health economists.

One final factor that has been subject to much discussion is the utilization of part-time medical personnel and voluntary personnel. There are considerable numbers of trained health workers who are not engaged in the health field. Many communities have developed programs to attract these people back into the active manpower pool by offering part-time and special shifts to accommodate them. This is especially true with regard to registered and practical nurses.

AVAILABILITY OF MANPOWER

Available health manpower is the actual supply of manpower at any given time. The national manpower supply is established by the interaction of supply components and utilization. The supply of manpower in any given area of the nation depends upon these two factors, as well as upon the national distribution of manpower.

Although much can be said in favor of simply creating a pool of manpower that is capable of meeting the medical needs of the nation, that alone is not enough. The next problem to be confronted is the distribution of manpower to those locations and occupations that have unsatiated demand (economic disequilibrium). It can be argued that the problems of manpower distribution and utilization are the real issues in the supply of health manpower. The utilization issue has already been touched upon. The following paragraphs will cover the distribution of manpower in the occupational and geographic sense.

Occupational Distribution: The problem of occupational distribution over-laps the discussion on utilization. The attempt to determine the best occupa-tional distribution to assure the delivery of health services is, thus, partially based on occupational definitions of who should do what, how many doctors are actually needed, etc. There is little more that can be said on the subject of distribution except that both occupational distribution and occupational definition are in need of a great deal of study. For example, why has the number of general practitioners declined from 120,000 during the depression years to 79,000 in recent years? And what has this meant to the delivery of health services?

Geographic Distribution: The geographic distribution situation is another problem. In 1971, there were over 130 rural counties in the United States that did not have a physician. The states of Alaska and Mississippi have only 69 doctors per 100,000 population, while New York has 199 per 100,000.[7] These problems exist because manpower is a resource that is difficult to distribute. Positive and negative location factors (city size, remuneration, racial distribution, available housing, etc.) influence the availability of man-power.[8] The distribution of four occupations, by state, and the rates per 100,000 population are listed in Table 3.

An increasing distribution problem is that of manpower by size of urban area. Tables 4 and 5 give an indication of the present physician distributions by city size. The very large cities of 1,000,000 or more tend to have the highest rates of physician manpower. It is interesting to note, however, that the rather small urban areas of 50,000 to 99,000 also have relatively high rates.[9]

When dealing with manpower data, the health planner must be careful in interpreting distributions and rates. Washington, D.C. is a good example. In 1970, there were approximately 3,023 physicians in the District of Colum-bia, or 318 per 100,000 population, engaged in the delivery of medical care. (The rest are involved in education, administration, research, etc.). The figure of 318 per 100,000, however, is deceptive. There are parts of North-

[7] Community Profile Data Center, Community Health Service. *An Analysis of the Current Status of Selected Health Manpower in the United States and Projections of Additional Re-quirements.* Washington, D.C., 1969.
[8] Acton, Jan and Levine, Robert. *State Health Manpower Planning: A Policy Overview.* Santa Monica, Calif., The RAND Corporation, 1971.
[9] Community Profile Data Center, *Analysis of Current Status of Selected Health Manpower in the United States.*

TABLE 3: SELECTED STATE MANPOWER LEVELS

State	December 1967 Non-Federal Physicians* M.D.&D.O.	Rate per 100,000	December 1966 Employed R.N.s	Rate per 100,000	December 1967 Active Physical Therapists	Rate per 100,000	December 1967 Registered X-ray Technologists	Rate per 100,000
Alabama	2,871	75	5,912	168	57	2	603	17
Alaska	177	69	590	223	21	8	55	20
Arizona	2,347	126	5,862	366	85	5	417	26
Arkansas	1,710	78	2,609	133	27	1	503	21
California	34,555	161	58,694	312	1,269	7	5,059	26
Colorado	3,685	168	8,312	425	140	7	934	47
Connecticut	5,422	164	15,438	536	205	7	1,128	39
Delaware	727	130	2,098	409	32	6	149	28
District of Columbia	3,023	318	3,662	454	133	17	154	19
Florida	9,447	126	21,760	369	265	4	1,424	24
Georgia	4,558	93	6,956	156	90	2	865	19
Hawaii	1,002	133	2,334	321	54	7	159	22
Idaho	676	89	1,954	280	19	3	181	26
Illinois	14,996	125	35,552	330	426	4	2,916	27
Indiana	5,158	94	12,829	259	112	2	1,253	25
Iowa	3,298	105	9,981	362	127	5	880	32
Kansas	2,680	106	6,895	303	67	3	659	29
Kentucky	3,168	90	6,297	198	68	2	593	19
Louisiana	4,095	103	6,758	187	75	2	745	20
Maine	1,238	114	4,051	414	34	3	311	32
Maryland	6,374	152	10,005	277	136	4	866	24
Massachusetts	11,195	181	28,743	532	377	7	1,668	31
Michigan	12,643	131	23,441	277	298	4	1,972	23
Minnesota	5,414	136	14,441	404	171	5	1,515	42
Mississippi	1,768	69	3,670	157	33	1	311	13

Missouri	6,832	129	11,291	247	189	4	1,116	24
Montana	726	97	2,483	354	14	2	180	26
Nebraska	1,717	106	4,730	329	47	3	448	31
Nevada	477	100	1,060	246	21	5	125	28
New Hampshire	964	119	3,521	521	35	5	242	35
New Jersey	10,041	133	24,942	362	226	3	1,320	19
New Mexico	1,050	91	2,511	250	31	3	223	22
New York	40,646	199	74,280	408	718	4	3,401	19
North Carolina	5,168	92	12,126	244	165	3	915	18
North Dakota	585	87	2,114	329	23	4	170	27
Ohio	14,760	129	32,649	315	374	4	2,807	27
Oklahoma	2,940	106	4,650	188	76	3	530	21
Oregon	2,935	128	6,814	345	120	6	629	31
Pennsylvania	18,728	143	45,809	395	503	4	3,090	27
Rhode Island	1,433	152	3,673	409	47	5	259	29
South Carolina	1,111	76	5,625	217	57	2	503	19
South Dakota	575	80	2,089	308	25	4	203	30
Tennessee	4,497	104	6,755	175	73	2	729	19
Texas	12,571	106	20,167	188	370	3	2,444	23
Utah	1,365	118	2,347	233	41	4	226	22
Vermont	790	149	1,836	447	33	8	186	45
Virginia	5,183	105	11,511	258	146	3	912	20
Washington	4,725	136	11,361	374	207	7	794	26
West Virginia	1,870	94	4,707	260	40	2	399	22
Wisconsin	5,218	112	14,084	338	246	6	1,536	22
Wyoming	322	95	1,209	379	11			37
USA	289,456	132	613,188	313	8,159	4	48,707	25

* Excludes: 27,724 federal physicians

Source: *An Analysis of the Current Status of Selected Health Manpower in the United States and Projections of Additional Requirements.* Washington, D.C., Community Profile Data Center, Community Health Service, March 1969.

east Washington—one primarily black community in particular—where the rate is 27 physicians per 100,000 residents.[10] (Tables 3, 4, and 5 in this chapter list total physicians and rates of physicians engaged in patient care.)

The discussion thus far has been an enumeration of the factors involved in the manpower system. No effort has been made to indicate a constructive approach to either manpower planning or estimating health manpower needs. The remainder of this chapter, however, will center on specific parts of the health manpower issue and the methods that may be used to deal with manpower problems.

PROJECTING MANPOWER NEEDS

Two of the most difficult problems of health manpower planning are defining and forecasting the future demand for care and, hence, the demand for manpower. The most common method of projecting health needs has been to consider the current utilization rate of the delivery system and, then, to use that rate as a standard for projecting future needs. To change the projection, one only needs to assume a different standard of medical care.

The disparity in projecting medical needs (and, hence, manpower needs) can be noted in the projections of physician manpower needs shown in Table 6. The dissimilarity in these projections is due, largely, to the inability to predict either the future mode of health care delivery or the standard of medical care that is to be achieved. It is interesting to note that the majority of projections have historically shown doctor shortages. All too often, however, it appears that projections have been produced to support policies that are beneficial to their promoters.[11]

It is not the purpose of this chapter to develop a model for projecting the future manpower needs of the nation. Rather, due to the inherent problems involved in making projections, the emphasis will be placed on influencing and manipulating the manpower now available to meet health needs. It is more important to understand the mechanisms that produce the supply of, and demand for, health services and manpower than to indulge in projections.

10 Richardson, Elliot L. "Meeting the Nation's Health Manpower Needs." *Journal of Medical Education,* 47(1):3–9, January 1972.
11 Hansen, Lee. "An Analysis of Physician Manpower Projections." *Inquiry,* 3(1):102–113, March 1970.

TABLE 4: MEAN NUMBER OF PHYSICIANS AND MEAN PHYSICIAN RATES PER 100,000 POPULATION BY TYPE OF SPECIALTY IN METROPOLITAN AREAS, BY TYPE OF COMMUNITY

Size of Community	Total Physicians Private Practice		General Practitioner Private Practice		General Surgeons		Obstetricians and Gynecologists		Psychiatrists	
	Rate	Mean #	Rate	Mean #	Rate	Mean #	Rate	Mean #	Rate	Mean #
1,000,000 and Over	111.64	2766.90	30.86	764.83	10.61	262.97	8.69	215.37	7.16	177.47
500,000–999,999	99.67	691.81	28.47	197.61	10.19	70.72	7.71	53.53	4.70	32.61
250,000–499,999	91.81	303.28	28.16	93.02	9.38	31.00	6.64	21.93	3.64	12.02
175,000–249,999	95.21	199.09	28.31	59.20	9.31	19.46	6.99	14.63	4.37	9.14
100,000–174,999	84.87	111.73	26.39	34.74	9.47	12.47	5.96	7.85	3.22	4.24
50,000– 99,999	97.92	81.36	27.72	23.04	10.94	9.09	7.00	5.82	4.35	3.62

Source: *An Analysis of the Current Status of Selected Health Manpower in the United States and Projections of Additional Requirements.* Washington, D.C., Community Profile Data Center, Community Health Service, March 1969.

TABLE 5: PHYSICIANS BY SPECIALTY AS A PERCENTAGE OF ALL PHYSICIANS, BY SIZE OF COMMUNITY

Type of Specialty	Size of Community					
	1,000,000 and Over	500,000 through 999,999	250,000 through 499,999	175,000 through 249,999	100,000 through 174,999	50,000 through 99,999
General Practitioners	27.6	28.6	30.7	29.7	31.1	28.3
Internists	14.4	13.1	11.5	11.7	11.3	13.7
Pediatricians	6.1	6.1	5.6	5.9	5.6	6.3
Allergists	5.2	5.6	5.1	5.0	5.1	3.3
Dermatologists	1.7	1.5	1.7	1.7	1.6	1.7
Other Medical Specialists	1.3	1.3	1.0	.9	.7	.7
General Surgeons	9.5	10.2	10.2	9.8	11.2	11.2
Obstetricians– Gynecologists	7.8	7.7	7.2	7.3	7.0	7.2
Ophthalmologists	3.8	3.9	4.1	4.3	4.5	4.7
Otolaryngologists	2.4	2.3	2.5	2.6	2.7	3.1
Urologists	2.2	2.2	2.6	3.0	3.0	3.1
Other Surgery Specialists	5.7	6.6	6.9	6.6	5.8	6.0
Anesthesiologists	4.0	4.0	3.9	3.7	3.3	4.1
Psychiatrists	6.4	4.7	4.0	4.6	3.8	4.4
Radiologists	3.1	3.4	3.7	4.0	4.2	4.8
Pathologists	1.4	1.4	1.6	1.7	1.9	2.9

Source: *An Analysis of the Current Status of Selected Health Manpower in the United States and Projections of Additional Requirements.* Washington, D.C., Community Profile Data Center, Community Health Service, March 1969.

With a pragmatic approach to manpower, a change in status can be effected, and it is possible to deal with the major programs and implications on state and areawide levels instead of nationwide. Before leaving the national manpower level, however, it should be noted that health manpower has been the subject of considerable legislation, most of which has focused on manpower training programs. In this connection, it should be noted that the greater part of the training effort consists of grants to universities for the purpose of setting up programs to train specific categories of manpower. Some representative manpower legislation is contained in the following Acts; also, there have been a number of Manpower Reports by presidential and congressional committees. Listed here are the most significant Acts and Reports.

Manpower Legislation:
Manpower Development and Training Act (1962)
Vocational Training Act (1963)
Health Professions Education Assistance Act (1963)
Nurses Training Act (1964)
Allied Health Professions Personnel Training Act (1966)
Allied Health Professions Personnel Training Act (1970)
Health Training Act (1970)

Manpower Reports:
The Ewing Report (1948)
The Bane Report (1959)
Health Manpower, Report 323; U.S. Department of Labor (1966–1975)
National Advisory Commission on Health Manpower, *Reports* I and II
  (1967)

TABLE 6: SUMMARY OF PHYSICIAN* PROJECTIONS FOR 1975

Projection Study	Demand	Supplies	(−) Deficit (+) Surplus
1. Bane Committee Report	330,000	(a) 312,800	−17,200
		(b) 318,400	−11,600
2. National Advisory Commission on Health Manpower	346,000	360,000	+14,000
3. Bureau of Labor Statistics (1967)	390,000	360,000	−30,000
4. Public Health Service	(a) 400,000	360,000	−40,000
	(b) 425,000		−65,000

Sources:
> Line 1—Surgeon General's Consultant Group on Medical Education. Frank Bane, Chairman. *Physicians for a Growing America.* Washington, D.C., U.S. Government Printing Office, 1959.
> Line 2—National Advisory Commission on Health Manpower. *Report*, Vol. II. Washington, D.C., U.S. Government Printing Office, 1967.
> Line 3—U.S. Bureau of Labor Statistics. *Health Manpower 1966–1975, A Study of Requirements and Supply.* Washington, D.C., U.S. Government Printing Office, 1967.
> Line 4—U.S. Public Health Service. *Health Manpower, Perspectives 1967.* Washington, D.C., U.S. Government Printing Office, 1967.

* Physicians include both M.D.'s and D.O.'s, except for Line 2, which excludes D.O.'s.

National health manpower efforts are simple in comparison to the planning and policy work of state and areawide groups. Although all must deal with a large degree of uncertainty that cannot be eliminated by better planning and analysis, the national health effort is not as directly concerned with health manpower as is the state or areawide agency. The state or area is faced with the problem of retaining its health personnel, while most health personnel remain in the nation; the state or area must attract manpower from other states and areas, while the national government is experiencing a gain in manpower through migration. The states have direct control of, and investment in, training facilities and schools, while the national government only subsidizes programs on an interim basis.

The state or areawide approach to health manpower planning should be a short- to intermediate-range function that surveys possible methods and policies to cope with uncertain manpower needs. This approach is substantially less satisfactory than full control and precise prediction; however, since these are impossible, such a method is realistic. Following an explanation of the state approach to health manpower, an overview of the actual manpower policy and planning of the 314(a) and 314(b) agencies will be given.

Health manpower problems vary from state to state and tend to be as complex as the states themselves; also, the factors causing the problems tend to vary as well. Following are some examples of these changing factors.[12]

1. Increased specialization in medicine has decreased the number of family physicians.
2. The average age of our population is increasing, thus shifting the health needs of the nation.
3. Educational institutions are overtaken by growing populations.
4. The emphasis on environmental health has increased the demands for health personnel.
5. Prepaid insurance, Neighborhood Health Centers, and Health Maintenance Organizations have increased the demands for health services.
6. Distribution of professional health manpower does not conform to consumer needs.

[12] U.S. Department of Health, Education, and Welfare, Program Development Branch of Comprehensive Health Planning, Health Services and Mental Health Administration. *Planning for Health Manpower*. Washington, D.C., U.S. Government Printing Office, 1970.

The solutions[13] to these problems are just as varied and can include such items as:

1. Increasing recruitment of personnel for health jobs.
2. Coordinating resources for health training.
3. Increasing flexibility of training programs.
4. Retaining trained persons in the labor pool.
5. Reorganizing jobs to obtain maximum utilization of personnel.
6. Modifying patterns of distribution.
7. Creating new job categories.
8. Increasing support for training health manpower.

The method to be used in approaching these problems and selecting the best solution for them is outlined in the following steps:

1. Gather and analyze data on health manpower and on demand for health services.
2. Define the manpower problem facing the specific locality or area.
3. Establish goals and priorities for the given situation.
4. Evaluate the impact of alternative solutions.
5. Recommend the most pragmatic application of resources.

The method, in short, is to plan.

Manpower planning at a state or areawide level should result in a set of policies that will aid in providing needed health manpower. Because of the uncertainties involved in determining health and manpower needs, these policies must be flexible and of an intermediate range. Also, because of the extremely long lead times in training health manpower, it is necessary to engage in this intermediate- and short-range planning in order to affect the available manpower supply within a reasonable period of time.

To gain a better understanding of the factors affecting health manpower, several specific occupational categories will be discussed. The emphasis here is on determining those factors that hold the greatest potential for impact on the manpower requirements in any given area.

---

13 U.S. Department of Health, Education, and Welfare, Program Development Branch of Comprehensive Health Planning, Health Services and Mental Health Administration. *Planning for Health Manpower.* Washington, D.C., U.S. Government Printing Office, 1970.

Physicians: Physicians require a longer training period than all other types of health manpower. Since there is usually a 10-year lapse between the beginning of college and the end of residency for physicians, an increase in medical school enrollments will be necessary if, in the long run, the supply of doctors is to be increased. At best, increased medical school enrollments will begin to show results in five to six years and, therefore, will not resolve short-run physician shortages. State financing of medical schools is often expected to augment the supply of doctors within a state. There is little doubt that it does. A large percentage of doctors, however, do not practice in the state in which they were trained. Studies have shown that increasing the enrollments in state medical schools is a difficult, expensive, and usually ineffective way to increase the supply of doctors in a state.[14]

Other means must be used to attract and retain doctors, and these tend to be of the location/distribution type. In examining these, it becomes evident that physician location behavior is very complex. Although many variables have been studied in relation to physician location, there are two that seem most effective: remuneration, and proximity to medical school activity.

In his study of physician supply, Frank Sloan[15] discovered a positive relationship between income potential and physician location. This fact has often been suggested, but Sloan states that, if all other things remain constant [they rarely do], a 1-percent increase in earnings will result in a 0.29-percent increase in the supply of available physicians. He also found that physicians tend to locate where the income is constant with little variation over time.

The second factor that Sloan found had an impact on physicians' location was medical school activity in the area. A study by Lee and Wallace[16] supports this finding. Apparently, physicians prefer to be close to an educational environment.

There are a number of other factors that have been related to physician location. Among these are the population of a given area; desirability of an area in terms of urbanization; and professional opportunities, including hospital privileges and licensure. Other factors that could be included in this list are forfeitable loans to students and/or new physicians, subsidies to attract

14 Acton, Jan and Levine, Robert. *State Health Manpower Planning: A Policy Overview.* Santa Monica, Calif., The RAND Corporation, 1971.
15 Sloan, Frank Allen. "Economic Models of Physician Supply." Unpublished Ph.D. thesis, Harvard University, 1968.
16 Lee, M.L. and Wallace, R. "Demand, Supply, and the Distribution of Physicians." Paper prepared for Western Economic Association Meetings, Long Beach, Calif., August 21–22, 1969. Cited by Sloan.

and promote relocation, and the shortening of the length of required clinical training.[17]

Dentists: There are two basic variables that tend to relate to dentists: relaxing licensure requirements for out-of-state training, and expanding the in-state capacity of schools of dentistry. Little study beyond this has been conducted.[18]

Registered Nurses: Programs to attract and utilize nurses must concentrate on two distinct areas: participation and training. In 1970, about half of the 1,100,000 trained nurses in the United States were working nurses. The remainder either held other jobs or were not working. An attempt to increase participation by nurses will probably have to be a hospital-based effort, since the shortage itself is hospital-based. The approach will have to include refresher training, special accommodations for part-timers, and day care for the children of working nurses.

Nursing education also needs updating. The scope of the nurse's job has changed significantly in the past decade. Emphasis on nonpatient duties often has been the reason for leaving the profession. Either new occupation categories will have to be created to make nursing more patient-oriented, or nursing schools will have to change their educational orientation to account for this.[19]

Allied Health Manpower: The allied health manpower supply is more susceptible to change through training than other fields are because it takes less time to train the allied professionals, and they tend to be less migratory than physicians. These professions also show a positive response to remuneration. Concomitant with growth has been the problem of recruiting people to enter these fields. Since few states presently utilize returning military medical corpsmen, it is very possible that the first states that will accept these veterans, recognize their abilities, and license them, may be in for a flood of medical personnel.[20]

---

[17] Acton, Jan and Levine, Robert. *State Health Manpower Planning: A Policy Overview.* Santa Monica, Calif., The RAND Corporation, 1971.
[18] *Ibid.*
[19] *Ibid.*
[20] *Ibid.*

MANPOWER PLANNING IN THE 314(A) AND 314(B) AGENCIES[21]

A 1970 study[22] of the state and areawide health planning agencies indicated that manpower was a problem of widespread interest. A large percentage of the agencies had specific groups working on the problem (see Table 7). The characteristic organizations for dealing with the problem were: a committee, a task force, or a contracted agency (that is, consultant, local university, etc.). In a few cases, the problem was being considered by the entire agency staff and advisory board.

The first manpower problem that most of the agencies encountered was lack of data. Although HEW and the Department of Labor have some data available, generally there is a lack of good data sources at the state and areawide levels. The 314(a) and 314(b) agencies attacked the problem in two basic ways: they gathered the data themselves or they contracted the job out. Some of the specific methods used were to:

1. Develop a joint library of data with Regional Medical Programs.
2. Cooperate with universities and industry using such data.
3. Conduct annual surveys.
4. Cooperate with other state and local agencies.
5. Hire a consultant or firm to develop the data.
6. Establish an ongoing data bank in the agency.

The specific health manpower problems that the agencies were faced with seemed to fit into seven broad categories, which were to:

1. Coordinate and expand existing training resources.
2. Expand school curricula and training resources.
3. Establish new training programs.
4. Promote health career opportunities.
5. Promote manpower utilization and productivity.
6. Recruit and retain health manpower.
7. Plan to alleviate physician, nurse, and dentist shortages.

It is evident from this short survey of planning agencies, as well as from this entire chapter thus far, that manpower planning is primarily a policy

21 U.S. Department of Health, Education, and Welfare, Program Development Branch of Comprehensive Health Planning, Health Services and Mental Health Administration. *Planning for Health Manpower.* Washington, D.C., U.S. Government Printing Office, April 1970.
22 *Ibid.*

TABLE 7: SUMMARY OF COMPREHENSIVE HEALTH PLANNING AGENCIES' INVOLVEMENT IN MANPOWER PLANNING*

	Number of Agencies	Number Recognizing Manpower Problem	Number Having Pertinent Committees or Task Force	Number Producing Pertinent Reports of Studies		Number Marketing Pertinent Recommendations	Number Developing Pertinent Legislative Proposals
				Completed	Under Way		
State 314(a)	50	48	41	18	17	16	3
District of Columbia and Territories 314(a)	6	6	2	1	1	2	0
Areas 314(b)	113	106	67	18	26	17	2

Source: *Planning for Health Manpower.* U.S. Department of Health, Education, and Welfare, Program Development Branch of Comprehensive Health Planning, Health Services and Mental Health Administration. Washington, D.C., U.S. Government Printing Office, 1970.

* This data reflects information available in the middle of fiscal 1970.

planning activity. Most planning is designed to meet state, regional, or local problems with specific programs or policies to fit the current perception of the manpower problems. In many cases, this approach is strictly pragmatic, but it is producing positive results.

SYSTEMS APPROACH TO MANPOWER

A number of fairly sophisticated models have been developed to predict manpower needs. There have also been models that have attempted to develop optimal mixes of technology and manpower. These are beyond the scope of this chapter, as they tend to be highly theoretical and quantitatively involved. There is, however, a systems approach that has promise for dealing with the manpower problem.

This approach was developed for use by the New Health Careers Demonstration Project and has been discussed in an article by Wilbur Hoff.[23] The objectives of the approach are: to improve the delivery of health services by restructuring health tasks and creating new careers; to design training programs for these careers in connection with health agencies, universities, and other community resources; to recruit and train persons for these career positions; and to determine the impact of this approach upon the delivery of health services to the community. This approach is institution or agency oriented and may be used for hospitals, neighborhood health centers, family planning agencies, nursing homes, etc.

The procedure involved is as follows:

1. Identify the agencies' health objectives.
2. Determine the changes that must be made in the population or environment to achieve optimization of the objectives.
3. Identify the tasks that workers must accomplish to achieve the desired change.
4. Analyze the tasks to develop job descriptions, to determine training requirements, to develop evaluation procedures, and to establish recruitment and selection procedures.
5. Restructure the tasks into new career ladders based on complexity, levels of responsibility, and training.

[23] Hoff, Wilbur. "Resolving the Health Manpower Crisis: A Systems Approach to Utilizing Personnel." *American Journal of Public Health, 61*(12):2491–2504, December 1971.

Once this procedure has been accomplished, training programs should be set up and accredited (if possible). Ideally, the persons recruited will be hired by the agency and given released time for training. The eventual result of the program may lead to new professional associations, certifications, and occupational recognition for the new careers developed.

The final stage of the program is the implementation of evaluations for the training programs and the effects of training on employers, on agencies, and on delivery of health services. Evaluation of these factors is an ongoing process that will allow the program and the projects to be updated as the health objectives of the agencies and the health needs of the community itself change.

SUMMARY

Health manpower is one of the most complex and difficult parts of the overall health system to deal with. To a large extent, this is due to the fact that manpower is a human resource which does not lend itself to allocation, as do land or capital. This fact forces the manpower planner to develop a series of policies that are flexible, yet deal with those factors that affect the manpower supply. In most cases, the policies will deal with methods for relocating the present supply of physicians, reactivating a large supply of nonworking nurses, and retaining as well as educating allied health workers.

REFERENCES

1. Robbins, Anthony. "Allied Health Manpower." *Inquiry,* 7(1):55–61, March 1970.
2. Schaefer, Morris and Hilleboe, Herman. "The Health Manpower Crisis: Cause or Symptom?" *American Journal of Public Health,* 87(1):6–14, January 1967.
3. Shuman, Larry; Young, John; and Naddor, Eliezer. "Manpower Mix for Health Services: A Prescriptive Regional Planning Model." *Health Services Research,* 6(2):103–119, Summer 1971.
4. Theodore, C. N.; Sutter, G. E.; and Haug, J. N. *Medical School Alumni, 1967.* Chicago, American Medical Association, 1968.

5. U.S. Congress, House Committee on Interstate and Foreign Commerce, Subcommittees on Public Health and Welfare. *Hearings on HR 16808 and HR 13100, Allied Health Professions Personnel Training: 1970.* Washington, D.C., U.S. Government Printing Office, 1970.

6. U.S. Congress, Senate Committee on Labor and Public Welfare, Subcommittee on Health. *Hearings on S. 3586, S. 2573, and S. 3718, Health Training Act of 1970.* Washington, D.C., U.S. Government Printing Office, 1970.

7. U.S. Department of Health, Education, and Welfare. *Health Manpower Source Book: Section 21, Allied Health Manpower, 1950–1980.* Washington, D.C., U.S. Government Printing Office, 1970. Public Health Service Publication No. 263, Section 21.

8. U.S. Department of Labor. *Occupational Manpower and Training Needs.* Washington, D.C., U.S. Government Printing Office, 1971. pp. 25–29. Stock Number 2901–0656.

9. Yett, Donald E. "Causes and Consequences of Salary Differentials in Nursing." *Inquiry,* 3(1):78–99, March 1970.

10. Steel, Henry B. and Rimlinger, Gaston V. "Income Opportunities and Physician Location Trends in the United States." *Western Economic Journal,* 3:182–194, 1965.

9

DETERMINATION OF REQUIREMENTS

The next step in the planning process is to determine the requirements of the community in order to meet its particular objectives. At this point, however, it should be remembered that planning is not a simple process, accomplished step-by-step in rigid sequence; but, rather, it is a process that often has many loops doubling back to earlier steps. For example, if the goal is delivery of adequate health services, objectives might very well have to be modified after the requirements of the community have been analyzed.

SOURCES OF INFORMATION ON REQUIREMENTS

There are three sources of information that may be used for assaying health requirements. These are: providers of care, consumers, and systematic analyses of data.

Providers of Care: This is the source most commonly used. It must be recognized that the viewpoints and inputs of the providers of care are influenced by a variety of things, including professional biases and, in some cases, even self-interests.

Consumers of Care: The second source is consumers of care. These people, however, are inclined to be nonsystems oriented. They tend to look at immediate problems rather than toward longer range effects or underlying situations. For example, it is entirely possible that consumers will emphasize care of the sick rather than prevention of illnesses.

Systematic Analyses of Data: The third source—systematic analyses of data—is a function of planners, whether they are employed by a planning agency or are members of an institution or service agency. Data, as it is regarded in planning, is something like a thermometer; it will tell you the level of a particular phenomenon, but, as with a clinical thermometer, if something is to be done with the data, then there must be a diagnosis that requires much more insight. This is why the planner, whoever he may be, has such an important role: because, in actuality, he is the diagnostician. For example, a community's morbidity rate may change, but this change may be the result of some population movement rather than the result of a health services program. The accuracy of such a diagnosis does not come solely from objective data, but is a function of the planner's understanding of the need perceptions of both providers and consumers.

DATA FOR DETERMINATION OF REQUIREMENTS

Regardless of the initial source of information on health requirements, data will be needed at least to validate the stated requirements of consumers or providers. As health needs receive higher priority, it may be expected that determinations will be based more and more upon objective evidence. Unfortunately, there is virtually no place today where one can find a complete health data system. The result is that most requirements are based upon data collected by a variety of agencies. This leads to some sizable problems that can be subsumed under three headings: accuracy, comparability, and focus.

Accuracy: The accuracy of data collected by other agencies must always be suspect. The user should ask questions concerning the completeness of the data and the exactness of the auditing to ensure that the collected data are valid. Remember, also, that what might have been adequate for the originator of the data-collection effort may not be adequate for the purposes of health planners.

Comparability: Comparability requires consideration of such issues as standard definitions and terminology, a common time frame, and identical boundaries of the geographic space covered. With regard to definition, problems occur in such areas as categories of patients. For example, one institution may consider a pediatric patient to be anyone from 0 to 12 years of age, whereas another institution may consider 0 to 16 years as the range of pediatric ages. With regard to time, it should be evident, for example, that 1967 morbidity data cannot be related to 1970 census data. With regard to boundaries, unless the area covered is the same, the data cannot relate to the same population. For example, health data may be collected by census tract, but a problem could arise if health data are used in conjunction with police data on arrests for drug abuse. This situation could occur because police data are collected by precincts, and precincts seldom, if ever, have boundaries coincident with census tracts or other geographic subdivisions.

Focus: The problem in regard to focus can be summed up by the term "small-area data." Health planners usually deal with a relatively small geographic area, or with communities or subareas. Unfortunately, most of the health data that have been collected officially are on the basis of very large samples, in fact, usually on a national level. Except to the extent that this gives a baseline or standard figure, which may be used as a point of comparison, such data are of little use to the planner. This is true because rates may vary from region to region, and absolute amounts may not be evenly distributed. For example, in one study of New Haven, Connecticut, it was found that even within census tracts where the population was not heterogeneous, there were substantial differences in infant mortality rates among block groups.[1] Another example, at a different level of analysis, is that it does not take much imagination to realize that national rates pertaining to the incidence of diseases associated with a certain industry, such as mining, are of virtually no use to local planners. Estimates that are based on the national average overstate the amount for those communities without mining industry and understate the amount for those communities that do engage in mining. Conversely, even when rates are identical, absolute amounts will vary with the density of the affected population.

SOCIAL INDICATORS

There have been some attempts to develop social indicators or a single health index to measure the health status of a community; to date, these efforts have

---

[1] U.S. Bureau of the Census. *Census Use Study: Health Information System II, Report No. 12.* Washington D.C., 1971. pp. 83–89.

been uniformly unsuccessful. Therefore, certain specific problems must be considered. One of major importance is that no general theory of health status that is analogous to the theory of national income or to the monetary theory of the economists has been advanced. A second problem concerns social goals. Often there is no general agreement on these goals, as there is on such economic goals as stability of prices and full employment. A third problem is the lack of a good theory of social causality, so that we do not really know what should be measured. For example, how much of a change in the health index could be attributed to a health program and how much to a rise in disposable income? And, finally, there is a problem of measurability. Many of the things that are considered important in the health field are intangible. Certainly, good health is more than just the absence of disease. At this point in the discussion, it should be emphasized that the state of the art is such that there seems to be no immediate prospect for developing suitable social indicators, insofar as good health is concerned; however, if a social indicator is to be used, then it must be scalable, reliable, and valid.

Scalability implies an ordering of outcomes, at least on a relative scale. As noted above, there is as yet no general agreement on health priorities.

Reliability means that the index would not be subject to measurement errors. Mortality data are generally considered to be quite reliable, although there are some cases of unreported deaths. Unfortunately, death, or the absence of death, is much too gross a criterion for measurement of health status in a developed country. When we turn to the alternative of morbidity data, however, we find that such data are much less reliable: first, because there is no systematic reporting of many illnesses and injuries; and, second, because there is a lack of standardization in nomenclature.

Validity implies that the indicator and the phenomena it is to measure must be highly correlated and, as pointed out above, that there is little empirical evidence on which to base a theory of the causation of health.

Since formal measures of health status are not currently available, we must rely on the crude proxies that have been used for many years. Often these were—and still are—used without a real understanding of their implications. For example, if one were to use the number of school days missed as a proxy, this index could be improved just as much by sending sick children to school as by eliminating the incidence of illness.

NEED OR DEMAND

Regardless of the measures used to determine health status, there is an underlying consideration that pervades all decisions concerning the establishment of health requirements, and that is whether the requirements should be planned on the basis of demand or on the basis of need.

DEMAND

If we plan on the basis of demand, it must be realized that the consumer demands only that which is economically rational for him to buy. Economic rationality, however, is not equivalent to health rationality, because there are certain situations in which other factors will have an overriding effect. The following are three demand situations. First, when an individual is suffering from great discomfort or feels that his life is in jeopardy, he is not likely to consider what the long-term effects of the necessary health care expenditures will be on his economic well-being. Second, demand is influenced by factors such as the type of service (life saving, cosmetic, or preventive), the price of the service, the educational background of the consumer, the consumer's race and ethnic background, the consumer's income, and the sex of the consumer. Finally, it is important to note that demand for health services is a derived demand. This demand, in nearly all cases, is modified by the dictates of the physician; it is also influenced by payment arrangements and, in many other cases, by the availability of the service. To illustrate the concept of derived demand, one must consider the patient who wants relief from certain symptoms. The services required to achieve this relief are determined by the physician, and, thus, the demand is derived. This derived demand may be for laboratory tests, X-ray examinations, drugs, etc.

NEED

The alternative to the demand situation is to project on the basis of need. Requirements generated on this basis represent the amount of health care that professionals believe is necessary. This is in contrast to demand, which is the amount of care that is actually used. There are two particular problems with need as a basis for a statement of requirements. First, the individual may not agree with the professional's determination of what his needs are. For example, the individual may have religious scruples against immunization. In this case, the need will exceed the amount that will ever be demanded. There is also the possibility that some individuals may perceive a need for health care in excess of what the medical community may consider necessary. An example of such need would be the annual physical examination of teen-aged children. In circumstances of this nature, the demand would again be different than the need, although it would be in excess of the need. It appears likely, however, that the number of such cases will be relatively small. Second, statements of need established on a professional basis do not consider the economic factors involved, especially the consumer's income level and his alternatives for spending that income. Thus, it is most likely that at any price above zero, the demand will be substantially less than the need identified by professionals.

NEED VERSUS DEMAND

To summarize the foregoing, need will lead to the identification of requirements that demand would overlook, but it may also lead to the development of services that consumers will not accept. On the one hand, need can lead to inflated statements of requirements by professional providers; need will not develop a scheme for rationing scarce resources among competing uses; people often need care before they demand it, in particular, they may need preventive services before symptoms or signs of need are perceived; and, similarly, many people who need care demand none or, at best, not enough. On the other hand, demand would overlook many important services because of consumer ignorance or misinformation.

The diagram in Figure 7 relates to services versus price, depicting a state of balance between what providers supply and consumers demand in keeping with traditional economic theory; but it has an additional line, NN, representing need. This depiction was developed by Jeffers, Bognanno, and Bartlett.[2]

In this diagram, the vertical line, NN, represents the quantity of services needed as determined by professionals. DD is a typical demand curve, and SS is a supply curve. The intersection of DD and SS determines the quantity demanded and the price required to attain equilibrium between supply and demand. In an equilibrium situation, there are no market shortages. (A market shortage may be defined as the difference between the amount that would be supplied and the amount that would be demanded.) But, there

---

[2] Jeffers, J.R., Bognanno, M.F., and Bartlett, J.C. "On the Demand versus Need for Medical Services and the Concept of Shortage." *American Journal of Public Health,* 61(1):46–63, January 1971.

would still be a need shortage—which is the difference between what people would demand at price P and the absolute amount of need, as determined by the professionals, without regard to economic considerations. The distance CN on the diagram is very interesting when considering the possibilities of national health insurance. In this case, the out-of-pocket price of health services might be zero, but there would still be a need shortage of the distance CN. This represents the effect of cultural, educational, and other influences that prevent the consumer from accepting all of the needed services even when they are free.

There are ways of shifting the demand curve to close the need gap; they include increasing the income of the consumer and, at the same time, subsidizing the cost of services, as done by Medicare and Medicaid. Also, education will have a primary role in shifting this demand curve. It should be noted also that a shift in the demand curve to the right will raise the equilibrium price as well as reduce the need shortages. The way to overcome this difficulty is to influence the supply curve. Typically, this is accomplished when the supply curve is moved downward by providing for such subsidies as medical education and research.

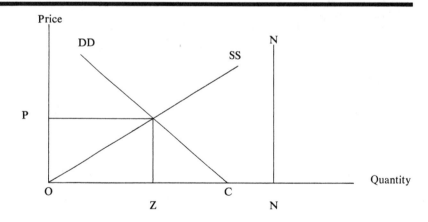

ON = Quantity of Medical Service Needed
OZ = Quantity of Medical Service Demanded and Supplied at P
OC = Quantity of Medical Service Demanded at Zero Price
ZN = Need Shortage of Medical Services at P
      (Quantity Needed—Quantity Demanded at Given Price)

Figure 7:   Need and demand for medical service

METHODS FOR DETERMINING REQUIREMENTS

Turning from these theoretical considerations that give us a broad background with which to conceptualize the probable outcome of whatever actions are taken, let us now look at some of the usual methods for developing health services requirements.[3] The first two of these, morbidity and mortality, are based primarily upon a need approach. The third, utilization, is a demand type concept.

MORBIDITY PROCEDURE

In order to use morbidity data, the community must be surveyed to find out what types of illnesses and injuries are experienced. This is necessary because, as stated earlier, there is no systematic reporting of all morbidity data. There are instances in which certain diseases are reported, and others in which case registers are maintained; however, these tend to be the exceptions rather than the rule. Once some sort of morbidity data has been obtained, the next step is to have professionals estimate the resources that are needed to cope with the level of morbidity that has been discovered. This is particularly difficult because it implies a requirement to aggregate needs based on different conditions of morbidity. For example, appendectomies have resource requirements that are very different from those for cancer.

MORTALITY PROCEDURE

Mortality data are more reliable and are much more readily available. With the exception of a few cases in which people make a conscious effort to avoid the normal disposition of the remains, the vital statistics system will record all cases of deaths. As with morbidity data, professionals must estimate some ratio or relationship between the level of mortality and the health resources required. It is obviously quite difficult to do this, because there can be a substantial amount of illness that does not cause death. Even when an illness is connected with death, the length of time and the amount of treatment involved vary widely among the various causes of death.

UTILIZATION APPROACH

Utilization data, as noted earlier, are based on the concept of demand rather

---

[3] Navarro, Vicente. "Planning for Distribution of Public Health Services." *Public Health Reports, 84*(7):573–581, July 1969.

than on need, but here a question remains concerning the relationship between supply and demand. It is often stated that the supply of health services creates its own demand; that is, if hospital beds are available, doctors will tend to fill them. Demand can be estimated by the extrapolation of current use data in the area or inferred by data from a similar area. This can be done by simple extrapolation, or it can be based upon a more complex multiple regression analysis. Utilization assumes that there will be no changes in technology or patterns of use, but this is certainly a dangerous assumption when one considers the great emphasis that is now being placed upon changing the methods of health services delivery. One way to avoid this dilemma is to provide the decision maker with a range of possible outcomes, and let him make a choice of the most probable outcome on the basis of subjective probabilities. Thus, if one were projecting the requirements for 1980, a three-level projection might be made based upon these factors: an extrapolation of current utilization rates; an increase in utilization rate projection premised on the introduction of national health insurance; and a low-utilization projection based on the idea that much of the current inpatient treatment will be replaced by ambulatory care once the Health Maintenance Organizations (HMO's) have achieved widespread acceptance. It is important to recognize that the precision of the projection will be markedly improved by first estimating the requirements for segments of the population (for example, females between 19 and 30) and then aggregating these estimates, rather than by applying a uniform utilization rate to the entire population.

Figure 8 presents an example of a utilization-based determination of requirements for ambulatory services or physician visits. At the outset, the annual use rate for various services is determined by age and sex group. This rate can be obtained from sample surveys or from group practices where records of client encounters are kept. If such records are used, however, one must beware of unusual use patterns by group members. In particular, the data collector must consider whether or not the group members get all their services from the group; if this happens to be a prepaid group practice, do the group members have an unusually high utilization rate? Once the use rates have been determined, these rates can be multiplied by population values for each year. Unless one is willing to assume a constant rate of use with no shift in demand, it would be wise to adjust the visit rate by some amount that will probably have to be determined on a subjective basis.[4] In

4 Navarro, Vicente. "Methodology on Regional Planning of Personal Health Services: A Case Study: Sweden." *Medical Care,* 8(5):9, September–October, 1970.

Age-Sex Groups	t_0			$t + 1$		
	Number	Visit Rate	Visits	Number	Visit Rate*	Visits**
			MALE			
0–14	1,000	.54	540	950	.55	520
15–44	1,000	.85	850	1,030	.87	900
45–64	1,000	1.02	1,020	940	1.04	980
65 and Over	1,000	1.33	1,330	830	1.36	1,130
Total Male	4,000		3,740	3,750		3,530
			FEMALE			
0–14	1,000	.54	540	940	.55	520
15–44	1,000	1.02	1,020	1,040	1.04	1,080
45–64	1,000	1.19	1,190	965	1.22	1,170
65 and Over	1,000	1.49	1,490	940	1.51	1,410
Total Female	4,000		4,240	3,885		4,180
TOTAL	8,000		7,980	7,635		7,710

* Approximate annual increase of 2%.
** Rounded off to the nearest 10 visits.

Figure 8: Determination of physician visit requirements

the example (Figure 8), it is assumed that the use rate is increasing annually by 2 percent; consequently, even though the population of this community is declining, the number of visits does not decline as rapidly.

ESTIMATING INPATIENT FACILITY REQUIREMENTS

When dealing with inpatient care in contrast to ambulatory care, the issue becomes somewhat more complicated, because one must consider length of stay as well as frequency of admission or contact. Therefore, three approaches to inpatient facility requirements will be detailed here: Hill-Burton, discharge distribution, and bed utilization.

HILL-BURTON

A widely used approach to the computation of inpatient bed need is the Hill-Burton method. This method applies to a designated service area, and the results obtained are compared to the number of conforming beds within the area. Note, in particular, that it does not consider the geographic distribution of beds. (Nonconformance, which is discussed in more detail in Chapter 7, is determined on the basis of U.S. Public Health Service regulations. There are three categories of considerations: nonfireresistive building, inadequate fire or safety protection, and facility inadequacy for the functions to be performed.)

In the example of the Hill-Burton method shown in Figure 9, the current use rate is determined by dividing the annual patient days by the total population size. This use rate and the projected population are used to compute a projected daily census. This, in turn, is an input to determine the number of beds required at a specific occupancy rate. To this is added an arbitrary number of 10 beds. The rationale for this number is to provide some capacity to absorb peak levels of demand. It is merely a safety factor, which may or may not be included, and may be of any size that the decision maker chooses.

a. $\text{Current Use Rate} = \dfrac{\text{Patient Days}}{\text{Total Population}}$

b. $\text{Projected Average Daily Census} = \dfrac{\text{Use Rate} \times \text{Projected Total Population}}{365 \text{ days/year}}$

c. $\text{Projected Number of Beds Required} = \dfrac{\text{Average Daily Census}}{\text{Occupancy Rate}} + 10 \text{ beds, an arbitrary}$

   number.

a. $\text{Current Use Rate} = \dfrac{720,000 \text{ (Patient Days)}}{800,000 \text{ (Total Population)}} = .9$

b. $\text{Projected Average Daily Census} = \dfrac{.9 \times 760,000 \text{ (Projected Total Population)}}{365} = 187$

c. $\text{Projected Number of Beds Required} = \dfrac{187}{.80} + 10 = 234 + 10 = 244$ (beds required
   at 80% occupancy rate.)

Figure 9:   Hill-Burton approach to the computation of inpatient bed needs

DISCHARGE DISTRIBUTION

The discharge distribution method, unlike the Hill-Burton method, applies to individual hospitals. This method is shown in Figure 10 and is explained as follows. Assume that there are three communities—X, Y, and Z. We are concerned with one hospital, Hospital A; therefore, for each community, we divide the number of discharges from Hospital A by the total discharges for the given period. This gives us a percentage of discharges. The percentage of discharges is then multiplied by the total population to determine the actual number of persons in that community who are served by Hospital A. This figure is then added for each of the three communities—X, Y, and Z—in order to determine that Hospital A is serving 90,000 people. To this is applied an arbitrary bed-to-population ratio in order to determine the number of beds needed. The weaknesses of this approach should be clearly evident to the planner, particularly the inherent problem facing him, that is, deciding what the bed-to-population ratio should be.

Community	Hospital A Discharges	Total Discharges	Percentage Discharges		Total Population		Population Served
X	100	300	33%	×	30,000	=	10,000
Y	200	500	40%	×	80,000	=	32,000
Z	400	500	80%	×	60,000	=	48,000
Total number of persons served by Hospital A							90,000

Figure 10:   Discharge distribution approach to inpatient facility requirements

BED UTILIZATION

A bed utilization method is shown in Figure 11. In this case, we estimate the number of admissions from the population, multiply this figure by the average length of stay, and thus obtain the number of bed days needed. Next, we

Estimated Number of Admissions × Average Length of Stay = Bed Days Needed.
8,000 Admissions × 9 days (Average Length of Stay) = 72,000 Bed Days Needed.
365 × Occupancy Rate = Days Available per Bed; or 365 × .8 = 292 Days Available per Bed.
Bed Days Needed ÷ Days Available per Bed = Beds Needed $\frac{72,000}{292} = 246$ Beds Needed

Figure 11:   Bed utilization approach to inpatient facility requirements

compute the days available for each bed, which is the average daily occupancy rate multiplied by 365 (days in a year). The number of beds needed is
determined by dividing the bed days needed by the days available per bed.

VARIABILITY OF ADMISSIONS AND UNIT SIZE VERSUS POPULATION

Each of the foregoing methods overlooked two important factors: first, variability in the rate of contact or the rate of admission; second, the relative size
of the population served. Both will be explained here.

EFFECT OF VARIABILITY OF ARRIVAL RATES

The first consideration deals with the variability of arrival rates over a period
of time. It requires a computation of the trade-offs between the use rate or
efficiency and the satisfaction of demand or effectiveness. Such a procedure
has been developed by P. J. Phillip,[5] and its adaptation and application to an
inpatient situation are illustrated in Figure 12. In this example, the trade-off
eventually must be made, with due attention given both to the capital costs of
additional service capacity and to the operating costs of unused capacity over
the life of the facility. Of course, the cash flow of the operating costs must be
discounted. To estimate this trade-off, the probability of each level of demand for service during a given period of time is first computed. This information can be obtained from records of the institution; but, in so doing, we
assume that there is some way to find out not only the amount of service
provided, but also the number of instances in which admissions were denied.
For example, if we were operating at a daily capacity of 300 units of service
and, on 182 days during the course of the year, the demand for service was
for 290 units, then the probability of a demand for 290 units of service
would be approximately .5. Similarly, if we found that the facility was fully
occupied, and that on 91 days 20 admissions were denied, then the probability of a demand for 320 units would be approximately .25. The first factor to
be computed, after we have determined these probabilities, is the average
number of daily services or, B, in Figure 12. Therefore, B is the sum of two
factors: the average utilization at levels below the hospital's capacity and

5 Phillip, P. J. "Some Considerations Involved in Determining Optimum Size of Specialized
Hospital Facilities." *Inquiry, 6*(4):44–48, December 1969.

average utilization based on full capacity. The first is computed by multiplying each utilization level below 100 percent by the relative frequency with which it occurs (percent of the time it happens). The second factor is computed by multiplying the hospital's total capacity by the relative frequency with which the hospital has had occupancy of 100 percent or greater. This latter step is necessary because it represents all those cases in which the total available resources were used, but, actually, the demand would be in excess of the available capacity. Once B has been determined, we can then compute C, which is the ratio of the number of services utilized to the number of services available. C is a measure of the effectiveness; H is the measure of efficiency.

Figure 12 shows three cases. In all three, the average daily demand is 110. In the first case, the number of beds available is 100; in the second case, 120; and in the last, 140. Obviously, B, which represents the average daily number of services used, does not increase proportionally with the size of the facility. Also, notice that as C increases, H decreases. It is the balance between C (the measure of effectiveness) and H (the measure of efficiency) with which the planner and the administrator must concern themselves.

Another method of determining the effects of variability in demand is described in the next section.

EFFECT OF UNIT SIZE

Turning to the second factor—size—there is a substantial difference in the outcome if we decide to put X number of beds in a single unit or to divide X number of beds among several units. This is a decision that involves serving a large population with one large unit or serving several smaller population groups with a number of smaller units. This difference is shown in Figure 13.

Essentially, the approach applies statistical theory by adding amounts equivalent to certain numbers of standard deviations to the average, in order to obtain a specified probability of meeting all demands for service. In this case, we are concerned with the level of demand for hospital beds and the average daily census. The standard deviation can be approximated by taking the square root of the average daily census.[6] Thus, if we want to be 95 percent sure of meeting the requirements, we can add the average daily census to 1.65 multiplied by the square root of the average daily census. The

[6] This is based on the assumption that the census data approximate a Poisson distribution, rather than a normal distribution.

$$B = \sum_{F=0}^{N} F\,PR + \sum_{F=N+1}^{\infty} N\,PR$$

$$C = \frac{B}{U}$$

$$H = \frac{B}{N}$$

| | | | N = 100 | | N = 120 | | N = 140 | |
			U = 110		U = 110		U = 110	
	F	PR	FPR	NPR	FPR	NPR	FPR	NPR
	80	.20	16		16		16	
	90	.20	18		18		18	
	100	.20	20		20		20	
	130	.20		20		24	26	
	150	.20		20		24		28
Total	550	1.00	54	40	54	48	80	28

$$b = 54 + 40 = 94 \qquad b = 54 + 48 = 102 \qquad b = 80 + 28 = 108$$

C = B/U = 94/110 = .85   C = 102/110 = .93   C = 108/110 = .98
H = B/N = 94/100 = .94   H = 102/120 = .85   H = 108/140 = .77

C Ratio of number of beds utilized to number demanded
H Ratio of number of beds utilized to number available
U Average daily demand for beds
N Number of beds provided
B Average daily number of beds used
F Daily demand for beds
PR Probability that F beds are demanded

Figure 12: Estimating trade-offs between service (C) and occupancy (H)

average daily census is computed by multiplying the number of admissions by the average length of stay and dividing the result by 365 (days in a year). In the example, we have taken an average daily census of 80 and, in the first part of the example, kept the 80 in one unit; in the second part of the example, we have placed it in two units. By centralizing this service, if we

Beds Needed $(P^* = .90) = ADC^{**} + 1.28 \sqrt{ADC}$

$\qquad (P = .95) = ADC + 1.65 \sqrt{ADC}$

$\qquad (P = .99) = ADC + 2.33 \sqrt{ADC}$

$$ADC = \frac{\text{Admissions} \times \text{Length of Stay}}{365 \text{ days per year}}$$

$$ADC = \frac{7300 \times 4}{365} = 80 \qquad\qquad ADC = \frac{3650 \times 4}{365} = 40$$

$$\sqrt{80} = 8.94 \qquad\qquad\qquad \sqrt{40} = 6.32$$

	Beds Needed	Occupancy Rate	Beds Needed	Occupancy Rate
P = .90	92	87	49	82
P = .95	95	84	51	78
P = .99	101	79	55	73

Comparison at P = .95

	1 unit	2 units
No. of Beds	95	102
Occupancy Rate	84	78
Daily No. of Unfilled Beds	15	22
Annual Cost @ $30 per diem (in thousands)	$164,000	$241,000
Annual Difference in Operating Cost	$77,000	

* Percent Level of Probability
** Average Daily Census

Figure 13:   Effect of size on occupancy rate

use the 95 percent level of probability, the number of required beds is reduced by seven, the occupancy rate is increased by 6 percent, and the daily number of unfilled beds is decreased by seven. Thus, at $30 a day, the annual cost of operating a single unit is $77,000 less than the annual cost of providing the same level of service with two separate units. This example applies particularly to certain specialized services, such as obstetrics, and makes a good case for consolidation of the OB services of several community hospitals.

REFERENCES

1. Falk, Shoshana. "Average Length of Stay in Long-Term Institutions." *Health Services Research, 6*(3):251–255, Fall 1971.
2. Gardner, Elmer A. "The Use of a Psychiatric Case Register in the Planning and Evaluation of a Mental Health Program." *Program Evaluation in the Health Fields.* New York, Behavioral Publications, Inc., 1969. pp. 538–561.
3. Gross, P.F. "Urban Health Disorders, Spatial Analysis and the Economics of Health Facility Location." *International Journal of Health Services, 2*(1):63–83, February 1971.
4. Hill, David R. "Hill-Burton Program—Planning Model Found Faulty." *Hospitals, 45*(24):46–50, December 16, 1971.
5. Karniewicz, Alfred J., Jr. "Estimating Coronary Care Bed Needs." *Hospitals, 44*(18):51–53, September 16, 1970.
6. Normile, F.R. and Ziel, H.A. "Too Many OB Beds?" *Hospitals, 44*(14): 61, July 16, 1970.
7. Siegel, Earl, M.D. et al. "Measurement of Need and Utilization Rates for a Public Family Planning Program." *American Journal of Public Health, 59*(8): 1322–1330, August 1969.
8. Wenkert, Walter; Hill, John G.; and Berg, Robert L. "Concepts and Methodology in Planning Patient Care Services." *Medical Care, 7*(4): 327–331, July–August 1969.

CHAPTER 10

COST-BENEFIT ANALYSIS:
A METHOD FOR EVALUATING ALTERNATIVES

When market conditions fail to produce approximately optimal results, then, inevitably, society will use nonmarket institutions to improve performance. There is wide agreement that performance in the health care field is considerably less than ideal. Therefore, the predictable result has been that government has become increasingly involved in the operation of this industry. For example, in 1970, public expenditures accounted for 37 percent of the national total outlay for health services.[1] Recently, in an effort to move toward its goal of reducing costs, the government has been placing heavy emphasis on improving the efficiency of the system. These improvements are being sought through many means, but the use of modern management techniques is being stressed. One of these techniques is cost-benefit analysis.

People in the health care field tend to resist such methods because they do not understand them, and they are uncomfortable with the new style of thinking that these techniques require; however, unless health care professionals learn these techniques, they will be unable to compete successfully for public support of health programs. Also, they will not be equipped to make the difficult, but necessary, choices among their own projects that are competing for the limited supply of funds allocated to health services.

There is ample evidence of weakness in this area. The Presidential Commission on Heart, Cancer and Stroke[2] estimated the benefit from cancer cure at $11.2 billion. In arriving at this figure, the Commission ignored the added costs of new treatment, assumed a sudden dramatic cessation in deaths from cancer, and made no effort to consider the time value of money. The National Conference on Medical Costs prepared a 322 page report[3] in which only one article, by Rashi Fein, even alluded to a relationship between costs

[1] U.S. Bureau of the Census. *Statistical Abstract of the U.S. 1971.* 92nd Edition. Washington, D.C., U.S. Government Printing Office, 1971. p. 62.
[2] Marshall, A.W. *Cost/Benefit Analysis in Health.* Santa Monica, Calif., The RAND Corporation, 1965. p. 3774.
[3] U.S. Department of Health, Education, and Welfare. *Report of the National Conference on Medical Costs, June 27–28, 1967.* Washington, D.C., U.S. Government Printing Office, 1968.

and benefits. A third example concerns a large, city health department which reported that it was contemplating a number of new public health projects. The criteria for selecting these projects seemed most unrealistic; apparently they sounded like good things to do, but the objectives showed an utter disregard for financial feasibility. For example, one project proposed to find *all* children with suspected heart disease or rheumatic fever. Think of the cost of finding that last child!

There is also good reason to believe that there will be increasing requirements for making difficult choices. Public Law 89–749, which includes the Comprehensive Health Planning Act, discontinued 16 categorical health grant programs and then replaced these programs with a single block grant for each state. The states now are forced to decide how to allocate these funds among the 16 programs and any other competing proposals as well. More recent legislation, authorizing revenue sharing among federal, state, and local governments, has increased the size and scope of choices that must be made at state and local levels. Further, there are proposals pending to make planning agencies responsible for the control of capital expenditures. All states have now established comprehensive health planning agencies at the state level, and the move to set up many counterparts at the local level is well under way. One group describes comprehensive health planning as a 10-step process. Three of the more important steps are to establish objectives, to formulate alternative means to attain the objectives, and to choose from among these alternatives. The third step is clearly a process in which the cost-benefit approach may be used. Whether one is working in a public agency at the national, state, or local level, or in a private institution, choices from among the alternatives must be made, and cost-benefit analysis is one effective approach.

Although early studies recognized the potential usefulness of cost-benefit analysis in the health field, very little effort was made to apply it until President Johnson issued his directive requiring all Federal Government agencies to establish a Planning-Programming-Budgeting-System (PPBS). HEW came to be considered the most successful user of this system outside of the Department of Defense. But even there, the number of studies was very limited because of the lack of qualified analysts; thus, HEW completed analyses of only 11 health-related programs. At state and local levels, use of this approach in the health field was even more limited. The most notable example of this technique was in New York City, where The RAND Corporation set up a PPBS for the Health Services Administration.

PPBS, as a total management system, is no longer being used by the Federal Government, but many of its components have been retained and are being used with increasing frequency. Cost-benefit analysis is one of the techniques that has survived, and it is flourishing.

As a result, there is a rapidly developing need for health care professionals whose skills include the ability to perform cost-benefit analyses. Further, all health care managers must have an understanding of this technique as it becomes more commonly used. Otherwise, they will become the captives of technicians who are competent in the technique, but who may lack knowledge and understanding of the health care profession. As an analogy, think of the number of crucial decisions that have been made by data system designers because top management was unwilling to learn the fundamental facts about computers.

PLANNING-PROGRAMMING-BUDGETING-SYSTEM (PPBS)

A brief history and description of PPBS, the context in which cost-benefit analysis emerged during the 1960's, may clarify both the purpose and methodology of cost-benefit analysis.

HISTORY

PPBS techniques apparently were first used by General Motors in 1924. They were "reinvented" by The RAND Corporation after World War II because of the need for data required by studies for the U.S. Air Force. These specialized skills, however, were generally ignored outside of The RAND Corporation until the Kennedy Administration, at which time they were adopted by the Department of Defense and received considerable publicity.[4] On August 25, 1965, President Johnson announced that PPBS would be put into use by all agencies of the Federal Government.[5]

This directive caused considerable furor. Efforts to implement PPBS varied from agency to agency and, because of a lack of obvious immediate success, enthusiasm waned. As mentioned earlier, PPBS is no longer being

[4] Novick, David. *Origin and History of Program Budgeting.* Santa Monica, Calif., The RAND Corporation, 1966. p. 3427.
[5] U.S. Congress, Senate Hearings Before the Subcommittee on National Security and International Operations, 90th Congress, 1st session. *Planning-Programming-Budgeting: Official Documents.* Washington, D.C., U.S. Government Printing Office, 1967.

used in its entirety by the Federal Government; however, many of its most important concepts and techniques remain, in other guises, as part of the Federal Government's armamentarium.[6]

DESCRIPTION

PPBS is comprised of two sets of complementary management techniques. It should be clearly understood, however, that either one can be used alone. The first half of this combination is program budgeting. A program budget has several distinct characteristics. It is structured by purposes rather than by objects of expenditures; for example, malaria eradication rather than salaries. Resource requirements are linked directly to the programmed outputs; that is, the amount of money to be spent on a particular program, such as control of a communicable disease, is made explicit. Finally, each program is projected far enough into the future to show its full cost rather than just the start-up costs that appear in the traditional budget. The second half of PPBS is cost-benefit analysis. This technique is used to aid in maximizing the difference between the benefit of a program and its cost by identifying the best alternative for carrying out the program.[7]

COST-BENEFIT ANALYSIS

HISTORY

Like PPBS, cost-benefit analysis is not really new. In 1844, a Frenchman, Dupuit, wrote a paper on the utility of public works. In this country, the River and Harbors Act of 1902 required the U.S. Corps of Engineers to select projects on the basis of benefits to commerce and the cost of these benefits.[8] Cost-benefit analysis currently is more widely used because of the development of operations research methods during and since World War II. The methods thus developed provided the necessary techniques; and the

---

[6] The reader who is interested in the details of these historical events could begin his research by scanning the indexes of *Public Administration Review* issued subsequent to 1964.
[7] Hitch, Charles J. "Decision Making in Large Organizations." In: U.S. Congress, Senate Subcommittee on National Security and International Operations, 90th Congress, 1st session. *Planning-Programming-Budgeting: Selected Comment.* Washington, D.C., U.S. Government Printing Office, 1967. pp. 10–17.
[8] Prest, A.R. and Turvey, R. "Cost-Benefit Analysis: A Survey." *The Economic Journal, 73*(4):683, December 1965.

increased availability of electronic computers has made their use feasible in everyday situations.

The use of cost-benefit analysis outside of the Defense establishment previously had received relatively little publicity. The Congress, however, has begun to take some interest in the possibility of applying cost analysis, both in its own decision-making process and, especially, as a requirement for receiving grants-in-aid. Such use would ensure that federal funds are spent wisely by nonfederal recipients.[9] The use of PPBS also has been endorsed by an impressive array of state/local government organizations, including the Council of State Governments, International City Managers' Association, National Governors' Conference, and the U.S. Conference of Mayors.[10] Recently, the George Washington University's State-Local Finance Project was engaged in a number of training and pilot operations designed to aid nonfederal governments in the implementation of PPBS. Also, individual institutions are beginning to use the technique of cost-benefit analysis in the selection of such things as computers and automated laboratory systems.

PURPOSE

In business and industry, cost-benefit analysis is analogous to capital budgeting. Both have the same problems, such as measuring benefits, establishing priorities, measuring the cost of capital, measuring intangible costs and benefits, and, ultimately, choosing the best of several competing proposals. In a more definitive vein, cost-benefit analysis is the systematic examination of alternative courses of action for a complex and uncertain future.

A systematic examination of alternatives is a radical departure from the requirements approach to budgeting. With this latter method, an agency would decide what it wanted to do and then would adjust its program to whatever size that could be supported with available funds. The requirements approach to budgeting, which focused on activity, often led to the selection of a program that offered very little improvement in relation to its cost. In comparison, the objective of cost-benefit analysis, that is, a systematic examination of alternatives, is to focus the analysis on a final output, which can

9 U.S. Congress, Joint Economic Committee, Subcommittee on Economy in Government, 90th Congress, 1st session. *Economic Analysis of Public Investment Decisions: Interest Rate Policy and Discounting Analysis.* Washington, D.C., U.S. Government Printing Office, 1967. p. 17.
10 Hatry, Harry P. "Criteria for Evaluation in Planning State and Local Programs." In: U.S. Congress, Senate Subcommittee on Intergovernmental Relations, 90th Congress, 1st session. *Planning-Programming-Budgeting: Selected Comment.* Washington, D.C., U.S. Government Printing Office, 1967. p. 12.

be produced in several ways. This can be difficult because the connection between inputs and outputs is not always well-known. It does, however, avoid building hospitals merely for the sake of having hospitals rather than for what they can do. The results of the Hill-Burton program might have been considerably different if this cost-benefit method had been available in 1948.

Because of complexities and uncertainties, there must be a large element of qualitative analysis, as well as the quantitative methods that are stressed in the literature. One of the dangers of using the cost-benefit method is that the analysts and decision makers may become so enthralled with the apparently neat answers it produces that they may forget about the simplifying assumptions that were necessary to arrive at that quantitative solution. Although all analytic techniques require simplification, the cost-benefit approach has virtues that the others lack. First, it offers a way of deriving numerical values that are logically consistent with one another and with the objective. Second, it accomplishes this by explicit processes that are open to critical evaluation or replication by others. In this connection, Alain Enthoven,[11] a leading proponent, stresses that cost-benefit analysis is neither occult nor synonymous with computers. A good analyst, he says, must be able to give a clear, nontechnical explanation of his methods and results to the responsible decision makers.

In short, as Fisher[12] says, cost-benefit analysis has a modest but significant role in decision making. Most major long-range decisions must be made on the basis of judgment, and the main purpose of analysis is to sharpen this judgment.

TYPES OF ANALYSES

This discussion, describing methods of analyses, will cover cost-benefit analysis, cost-effectiveness analysis, and benefit/cost ratio—a type that must be used with care.

---

[11] U.S. Congress, Senate Hearings Before the Subcommittee on National Security and International Operations, 90th Congress, 1st session. *Planning-Programming-Budgeting: Select Comment.* Washington, D.C., U.S. Government Printing Office, 1967. p. 2.

[12] Fisher, G.H. "The Role of Cost-Utility Analysis in Program Budgeting." In: Novick, David, ed. *Program Budgeting.* Cambridge, Mass., Harvard University Press, 1965. p. 67.

Cost-benefit analysis depends upon the scope of the comparison; it can be analyzed as intrasystem, intersystem, intraprogram, and interprogram.

Intrasystem analysis compares alternative methods for a given system; for example, movement of patients by helicopters versus movement by conventional ambulances.

Intersystem analysis compares alternative systems within a program; for example, a preventive medicine system versus a curative medicine system.

Intraprogram analysis compares alternative combinations of systems that are aimed at the same general objective; for example, to maximize health during an entire life span. This is sometimes called force structure analysis.

Interprogram analysis deals with competing goals, for example, health versus welfare.

The significant thing about this categorization is that a move from intrasystem analysis to interprogram analysis is accompanied by a gradual shift from very precise quantitative formulations to a much more qualitative mode of analysis. To some extent, this is due to the increasing complexity of the problem, but the major reason is the greater difficulty encountered in developing equivalent measures of the outputs. For example, it is not too difficult to compare time-lags in getting a patient to the hospital by various modes of transportation. But what are the relative values of eradicating lung cancer and of assuring that every citizen completes high school?

COST-EFFECTIVENESS ANALYSIS

This categorization involves the distinction between cost-benefit and cost-effectiveness. Although some of the original workers in the health care field see no difference between cost-benefit and cost-effectiveness,[13] most practitioners find it useful to make this distinction.[14] Essentially, in cost-benefit studies, both inputs and outputs are variable, while in cost-effectiveness studies, one of the two is held constant.

Cost-effectiveness is used to avoid problems of measurement. In analyzing health services for the poor, for example, HEW found that the many alternatives available were not mutually exclusive; thus, there could have been an infinite number of possible combinations. Consequently, HEW established a fixed budget for inputs and presented a limited set of output combinations to

[13] McKean, Roland N. *Public Spending.* New York, McGraw-Hill, 1968. p. 135.
[14] Crystal, Royal A. and Brewster, Agnes W. "Cost-Benefit and Cost-Effectiveness Analyses in the Health Field: An Introduction." *Inquiry,* *3*(4):4, December 1966.

the decision makers for choice. This is a rather unusual approach. In most cases, an attempt is made to determine the least-cost method of reaching a fixed level of output (for example, reducing the incidence of lung cancer by 10 percent). Because of the difficulty in assigning values to outputs, this approach is favored by practitioners, but it does have two disadvantages. First, it limits quantitative comparisons to the intrasystem level; that is, to the level where outputs are identical. Second, as Ackoff[15] points out, it simply shows which is the better of two alternatives. There is no guarantee that either one is optimal or even adequate; but, by holding constant either input or output, cost-effectiveness analysis keeps the user from falling into the trap of striving to maximize outputs and minimize inputs simultaneously. The cost-benefit method allows both to vary, but both cannot go to their extreme values at the same time.

BENEFIT/COST RATIO ANALYSIS

Benefit/cost ratio is another type of analysis, but it must be used with caution for it can be misleading. It is especially common in situations where monetary values cannot be assigned to outputs. Maximization of the ratio is considered the ideal, but, in actual fact, the ratio is irrelevant; the real question is whether the extra output is worth the added cost or whether the program is operating at the proper scale. For example, 20/10 ratio is numerically equivalent to 200/100; but it does not mean the same to the person concerned with the absolute level of accomplishment. It is interesting to note that, although many studies have used ratios as criteria, nevertheless, in the last analysis, decisions also were based on judgment regarding scale of programs and estimates of need.

STEPS IN ANALYSIS

A full systems analysis involves the following steps or phases: *One*, establish the objectives, define the environment in which these objectives will be sought, and develop alternative methods; *two*, determine the interrelationships among variables within the system and then construct models of the system; *three*, measure costs; *four*, measure benefits; and, *five*, document the analysis so that it can be re-evaluated, if necessary, and present the results in

15 Ackoff, Russell L. "Toward Quantitative Evaluation of Urban Services." In: Schaller, Howard G., ed. *Conference on Public Expenditure Decisions in the Urban Community.* Washington, D.C., Resources for the Future, Inc., 1963. p. 95.

terms suitable for the decision maker. Each of the first four steps will be discussed separately.

STEP ONE: OBJECTIVES, ENVIRONMENT, AND ALTERNATIVES

Establishing the Objectives: During this phase, the analyst must have an opportunity to work closely with the decision maker, or there is a great possibility that he will accomplish a feat of technical virtuosity that is utterly useless. Therefore, he must be sure that he is working toward the proper objective on the basis of acceptable assumptions with methods that are politically feasible. For example, despite the doctrine of sunk costs, decision makers are bound to some degree by what has happened in the past; thus, in many areas, substantial investments limit the courses of action that are practically available.

The most important characteristic of objectives is that they must be oriented to ends and not to means. This is not as easy as it sounds because, often, the end results are far less measurable than are the means. For example, a recent study concerning ambulance services—where the criterion was speed in getting emergency patients to the hospital—failed to show that there was any demonstrable relationship between speed and patient welfare. Also, the criteria used to measure attainment of objectives must be broad enough so that any unwelcome side effects of the proposal will be detected. For example, it is possible to reduce costs by failing to provide services (such as diagnosis and treatment), but the indirect costs (such as loss of productivity due to illness, disability, and debility) will continue. A side effect that is often overlooked in analysis, but which is tremendously important to public decision makers, is the redistribution of income. In a hospital setting, the analogous effect is a shift of charges from one group of patients to another.

Defining the Environment: Many of the assumptions about the environment are political in nature, and this leads to much criticism of the cost-benefit method. Many of the critics of cost-benefit analysis either do not understand, or do not believe, those statements about using analysis as a supplement to judgment in the decision-making process. They allege that analysts overemphasize efficiency without considering other consequences. In the words of a senator, ". . . the analysts emphasize crass materialism rather than American ideological values."[16]

---

16 U.S. Congress, Senate Hearings Before the Subcommittee on National Security and International Operations, 90th Congress, 2nd session. *Planning, Programming, and Budgeting.* Washington, D.C., U.S. Government Printing Office, 1968. p. 145.

A more rational critic insists that the analysis depends upon a prior political framework, but, within that framework, it can be very useful. This view is certainly supported by other writers, one of whom[17] suggests that the practitioner may well find Banfield's *Political Influence* to be just as important a book as Hitch's *Decision Making for Defense*. These words may reflect experience with the dental care program analysis. Fluoridation was shown to have a very high benefit-to-cost ratio, but it was replaced in the Johnson Administration's legislative proposal by a more expensive and less effective treatment program because of dread of the very vocal antifluoridites.[18] Actually, the analyst who ignores the political aspects of a program does so at his own risk. Few programs of any consequence can be initiated unilaterally, and the interests of other parties are very likely to cause modification of the pure proposal to such an extent that achievement of the expected goals is most unlikely.

Developing Alternative Methods: This phase can be mutually beneficial to both the analyst and the decision maker. Often, the decision maker does not have the time to develop alternatives on his own, and this leads to rigidities which are the hallmarks of bad planning. There is no single right way. Alternatives must be considered at every level of decision making, and cost-benefit analysis provides a more or less systematic method for defining and considering useful alternatives. For the analyst, it avoids the expenditure of effort required to develop a full study of alternatives that will never be seriously discussed.

STEP TWO: DETERMINE INTERRELATIONSHIPS IN THE SYSTEM AND CONSTRUCT MODELS OF ALTERNATIVES

Characteristics of Models: Once a set of alternatives has been selected, the next step is to construct models of these alternatives. These can be used to determine what the outcome of each alternative might be. A model is an explicit representation of some system or object. It includes the components, the interrelationships among the components, and the boundaries within which the system operates. Models have three important characteristics: abstraction, simplification, and substitution.

---

[17] Kissick, William L. "Planning, Programming and Budgeting in Health." *Medical Care*, 5(4):201–220, July–August 1967.
[18] Drew, Elizabeth B. "HEW Grapples with PPBS." *Public Interest*, 7:27, Summer 1967.

Abstraction. Because it is developed at a higher level of generality than the specific object or system, the model can be taken to represent the entire class or set of objects with which we are concerned.

Simplification. Closely related to abstraction, it deals with elimination of certain complexities that have very little influence over the operation of what we are modelling. For example, if we were modelling a multiphasic screening, it might not be necessary to include in the model the details of how the patient moved from one part of the unit to another. This illustration should make it clear that the kind and degree of simplification must depend upon the purposes for which the model is to be used.

Substitution. As stated earlier, a model uses other things (words, mathematical symbols, analog circuits) to represent the objects in which we have an interest.

Reasons for Using Models: The three characteristics described above form the basis for the various reasons for using models rather than dealing with the actual object. There are at least five of these reasons.

Cost Saving. Generally, it is much cheaper to use representations of the object than the object itself. For example, we cannot afford to build each of the alternative designs that might be considered for a health facility and then choose from among those completed facilities.

Time Saving. Very often the actual object or system operates at a relatively slow pace; therefore, it takes a long time before the impact of changes can be seen. Models can speed up the process by scaling down time. For example, if a model of a hospital admission system were being constructed, a computer simultation could easily produce the results of a year's experience in less than one hour.

Safety. Very often in the health field, our attention is focused on objects involving people. Models allow us to make preliminary estimates of what the effects of alternative courses of action might be without the risk of adverse effects on human beings, since representations are used in lieu of actual people.

Analysis. Building a model requires the designer to have a thorough understanding of all the components and the interrelationships. Thus, it forces him to obtain a clear conception of all that goes on within the real system.

Reproducibility. Because of the economies in time, money, and risk, it is possible for the original analyst to reproduce his model in such a manner as to make it feasible to examine a great many alternatives. In other words, it gives him a much wider range of choices in his analysis. Furthermore, it allows other persons, who enter the decision-making process at a later stage, to reproduce the model and to test the outcomes, using different inputs which their respective judgments deem to be better than those used in the original study.

Types of Models: There are many types of models, ranging from replica models—which look and function exactly like the real object—to symbolic models—which use abstract symbols (diagrams, mathematical equations, etc.) to represent the real object.

For our purposes, we are primarily concerned with the abstract, in which statistical or engineering models are developed to represent some component of a health care delivery system. Since these types of models typically involve mathematical equations, it should be noted that there are two possible forms of mathematical models: deterministic and probabilistic.

In the *deterministic model*, the relationship among components is considered to be fixed. For example, such a model might state that one pediatrician can care for 15 patients during a four-hour shift in an outpatient clinic. In the *probabilistic model*, it might be shown that the relationship among components will vary in accordance with some sort of statistical distribution.

In practice, it is possible to combine both probabilistic and deterministic components in a single model; but, when this is done, the outcome must necessarily be treated as that of a probabilistic model. In such cases, each run of the model is considered to be an individual experiment. It is necessary, therefore, to make many experiments and to take the mean value of the outcomes of these experiments in order to determine what the expected value for the real system would be.

Design of Models: Two approaches to the design of models will be considered. The first of these is the statistical approach and, the second, the engineering method. The statistical approach takes data from a large number of similar cases and then applies these data to estimate how the planned alternative would work. The data can be collected longitudinally—that is, for a few institutions over a long period of time—or on a cross-section basis—that is, from many similar institutions at a single point in time. The difficulty with the latter approach in the health field is that it is virtually impossible to find a sufficient number of similar institutions from which to gather an adequate set of data. On the basis of the longitudinal approach, we would have to assume that health institutions had not changed their methods of operation over many years; but we know that this is not the case. In terms of similarity among units at one point in time, we encounter the problem of differences in services offered among hospitals which, on the surface, appear to be quite similar. For example, there are three large teaching hospitals in Washington, D.C. Even though they may seem very much alike, it is entirely possible that the management of a particular type of surgery might vary substantially among the three. The resulting differences in resources used and in the assignment of costs would thus be significant.

The engineering method of model building assumes that the basic components of the object or system can be identified; also, that the relationships among them can be determined, so that a total structure can be built up from these individual parts. One of the first problems encountered is the level of detail to which these components should be broken down. For example, if we are dealing with a neighborhood health center, should the laboratory be treated as a single entity or should it be broken down into parts, such as chemistry and hematology? Frequently, the components and/or the functions within a unit are irrelevant or unknown. In such cases, we apply what is known as the black-box approach. Specifically, the black-box approach means that we concern ourselves simply with the input and the output from that component. For example, we might know that the assignment of 3 cooks, 2 bakers, and 12 dietary aides will allow us to produce all meals required for 300 inpatients during a seven-day week. If satisfactory data on the operation of the black box are not available in current experience, test results may be used as substitutes. The experimental operation is closest to reality and involves decision makers as actors in a real environment. Demonstration projects can be quite useful for getting data of this sort. Unfortunately, although demonstration projects are quite common in health care institutions, seldom do they make the effort to collect information on anything except the direct clinical aspects of the program.

STEP THREE: COST MEASUREMENT

Some of the most important economic concepts in cost-benefit analysis are the various types of costs and economies of scale. Unless the decision maker considers the proper cost, he will almost certainly make the wrong choice. Since cost-benefit analysis is oriented toward selecting future programs, it is probable that most alternatives will involve long-run costs based upon nearly complete variability of inputs. Thus, possibilities of increasing or decreasing returns to scale become highly significant.

Several types of costs that the health care practitioner is likely to encounter and that he must take into consideration when selecting future programs will now be discussed.

Opportunity Cost: This type of cost, which usually is not very well understood, should be used when the supply of some input is strictly limited. Essentially, opportunity cost is the potential value from some action that cannot be taken because all of the available limited resource is being used in other activities. If the value gained from one of these activities is less than the opportunity cost of any alternative, then the rational decision maker will feel obligated to discontinue that activity and substitute for it the most valuable alternative that is available. To explain this point, periodic physical examinations require many man-hours of physician effort, but there is no evidence that systematic screening detects a significant number of asymptomatic illnesses. Therefore, as long as the number of physicians is insufficient to provide all of the needed treatment, a program of widespread, complete physical examinations probably will not be able to pass the test of opportunity cost.

Sunk Costs: Those costs that will not be altered as a result of the decision being considered are known as sunk costs. Consequently, costs of this type are irrelevant. To determine whether or not any particular cost should be categorized as a sunk cost will depend upon the scope of the decision. For instance, ownership costs of a truck would be irrelevant in a decision relating to alternative uses for that truck, but they would be relevant in a decision involving alternative types of vehicles.

Incremental Costs: These are additional costs that result from a change in activity. Arising from a decision, they appear to be more relevant for decision making than are those average costs that include sunk costs. For example, a share of depreciation should not be included in the cost of going on a seven-day schedule in the operating room, since no additional facilities are required for this change in activity. In this type of situation, it is probable that the only significant relevant costs would be salaries.

Average Costs: These are total costs divided by total units of output. They frequently mask important differences. To explain this point, typical health care data are presented in terms of cost per patient day. A study of a domiciliary care program by Ingbar and Lee,[19] which used special cost collection techniques to avoid the usual aggregation and allocation that occurs in a hospital accounting system, clearly showed how misleading these averages can be. Occupational therapist and physician visits cost an average of $0.14 and $0.44 per day, respectively, for all patients; but when the focus was shifted to cost per day for patients using the services, the average costs for therapist visits became $0.52. Costs for physician visits remained the same.

Marginal Costs: These costs occur when one more unit is added. The Ingbar and Lee study demonstrated the importance of using marginal rather than average costs. As shown above, the average cost of a physician visit was less than the average cost of a visit by a social worker—in this case, an occupational therapist. Logically, the program director should substitute the former for the latter, since the physician could presumably perform most, if not all, of the functions of the social worker. Because of the limited supply of physicians, however, the marginal cost of adding physicians to the staff would surely be much higher than the average cost for physicians or the marginal cost for social workers. Consequently, a decision based on average costs for both physician and social worker visits would increase rather than decrease the total cost of the program.

This concludes the discussion on the various kinds of costs that must be considered by the health care planner in analyzing the cost-benefits picture. At this point, however, before proceeding to step four of the analysis, the problems relating to cost measurement and the long-run cost situation will be reviewed.

PROBLEMS OF COST MEASUREMENT

For many practical purposes, marginal costs and incremental costs are synonymous. A good technique for determining costs is to plot total cost as a function of the cumulative number of units produced. When this is possible,

[19] Ingbar, Mary and Lee, Sidney S. "Economic Analysis as a Tool of Program Evaluation: Costs in a Home Care Program." In: *The Economics of Health and Medical Care.* Ann Arbor, Mich., The University of Michigan, 1964. pp. 173–210.

it will provide total fixed cost, total variable cost, and marginal cost. It would be dangerous, however, to extrapolate beyond the observed data because these functions may not be linear. The use of this so-called accounting method of cost estimating is severely limited because virtually all available health cost data are collected in accounting systems that do not separate relevant costs from irrelevant costs (see pages 199–201). As mentioned earlier, the problems of incommensurability generally rule out the use of the statistical approach to these problems. Consequently, it appears that the engineering method of cost estimating has promise for the foreseeable future. The engineering method involves identifying all the components of a system, assigning a cost to each component, and then aggregating these costs to arrive at the total cost for the system.

LONG-RUN COSTS

The foregoing discussion is related primarily to the measurement of short-run costs, that is, costs of varying rates of output with a fixed level of plant or technology. In the planning process, interest focuses on the long-run costs that arise when all factors are variable. The long-run cost function can be visualized as an envelope curve enclosing short-run cost curves, each of which represents one of the feasible plant sizes (for example, number of beds in a hospital) or production techniques. It is especially useful in determining the optimum plant size and/or measuring the costs of using other than optimum plant size to achieve a desired distribution of locations. The data problems are particularly acute in the development of a long-run cost function because the estimates must be based upon comparable inputs and outputs for plants of many sizes. As noted earlier, this is nearly impossible in the health field at the present time.

STEP FOUR: BENEFIT MEASUREMENT

Many studies avoid the problem of benefit measurement by holding output at a constant level. By doing this, they drastically lower the level at which quantitative comparisons can be made. Thus, the measurement of benefits is an important phase in a full systems analysis study.

The value of human life and health has been under study since the efforts of Sir William Petty in the 17th Century, but there still is no widely accepted method for assessing this quantity.[20] One analyst set the value of an airplane

[20] Marshall, A.W. *Cost/Benefit Analysis in Health.* Santa Monica, Calif., The RAND Corporation, 1965. p. 2.

accident victim at $373,000,[21] while another analyst suggested that the appropriate value should be measured by the utility of risk avoidance to the target population.[22] Most studies that use dollar values, however, tend to follow the concepts outlined in Mushkin's landmark article, "Health as an Investment,"[23] which focuses on losses in productivity. To date, the most complete effort along these lines is Rice's *Estimating the Cost of Illness.*[24] It provides tables that give present values of expected future earnings for various age groups, by sex, as indirect costs of illness or death; it also provides data on expenditures for health care as direct costs of illness. It is unfortunate that the latter, for lack of a better alternative, were estimated for gross diagnostic categories on the basis of data that were derived from the Professional Activities Study (PAS). These data are the best available, but the participants in PAS are hardly a representative sample of all U.S. hospitals.

For benefit measurement, as for cost measurement, there are many problems to be dealt with, and a review of a few of the more significant problems that the health planner might encounter follows.

PROBLEMS OF BENEFIT MEASUREMENT

Measurement problems lie just below the surface in all of these methods. These include: how to handle taxes and transfer payments to avoid double counting; how earnings should be adjusted for possible future increases in productivity; whether it can be assumed that all people who avoid illness will be employed continuously in the future (for example, whether the possibility of an alternate illness or a decline in the national employment level should be considered); whether what a person who is saved from death consumes should be deducted from his gross earnings stream; and what earnings should be imputed to housewives or to children whose entrance into the labor force is delayed by illness.

Furthermore, there are the problems of measuring the unmeasurables. The following are just a few of the possibilities in this area. Klarman[25] asserts

---

21 Fromm, Gary. "Civil Aviation Expenditures." In: Dorfman, Robert, ed. *Measuring Benefits of Government Investments.* Washington, D.C., The Brookings Institution, 1965. p. 196.
22 Schilling, T.C. "The Life You Save May Be Your Own." In: Chase, Samuel B., Jr., ed. *Problems in Public Expenditure Analysis.* Washington, D.C., The Brookings Institution, 1968. pp. 127–176.
23 Mushkin, Thelma J. "Health as an Investment." *The Journal of Political Economy,* 70(5):129–157, October 1962.
24 Rice, Dorothy P. *Estimating the Cost of Illness.* Health Economics Series No. 6. Washington, D.C., U.S. Public Health Service, 1966.
25 Klarman, Herbert E. "Syphilis Control Programs." In: Dorfman, Robert, ed. *Measuring Benefits of Government Investments.* Washington, D.C., The Brookings Institution, 1965. p. 400.

that people will spend more to avoid, or to be cured of, a disease than the value of direct and indirect costs as computed by Rice. He proposes the technique of the analogous disease to estimate how much this will be. In his example, psoriasis is used as an analog to syphilis because it is not disabling, but it does have symptoms that people want to get rid of. If the cost of getting rid of the symptoms of psoriasis was $50, then this component of the cost of an episode of syphilis would be approximately $50. Weisbrod[26] argues that the distribution of nonmonetary costs (for example, sorrow over death) is approximately that of economic costs (that is, both costs are highest at middle life and least in infancy and old age). Hatry[27] suggests that a panel of experts could be used to rank alternatives subjectively when unquantifiable factors, such as amount of discomfort, are involved. Another benefit to the patient, which is usually overlooked, is the advantage of having alternatives from which he can make a choice. Too often, health care professionals are overly paternalistic, but how can the variety of choices be valued?

Finally, health programs are very likely to have definite effects on the distribution of incomes (for example, from a reduction in unemployment); therefore, it is important to show which regions or population groups will benefit, and, in the overall picture, just how much society will gain. This is a crucial issue in the political decision-making process. A vocational rehabilitation study that attempted to do this was particularly interesting, and the result established an important point. Ultimately, it demonstrated that reductions in welfare payments, plus taxes on income earned by those rehabilitated, would be two to four times greater than the tax cost of the program.[28]

ADJUSTMENT IN COST AND BENEFIT MEASUREMENT

In summing up steps three and four of a full systems analysis, it should be noted that, in most cases, both cost and benefit data must be adjusted for three factors: time value of money, price changes, and risk and uncertainty. The first type of adjustment makes it possible to compare projects having different life cycles and different patterns of cost outlay and receipt of benefits. The second factor is necessary in order to compare the monetary data collected during different periods. Since cost-benefit analyses are designed for

---

26 Weisbrod, Burton A. *Economics of Public Health.* Philadelphia, University of Pennsylvania Press, 1961. p. 96.
27 Hatry, Harry P. State-Local Finance Project, George Washington University, Washington, D.C. Interview on November 26, 1968.
28 U.S. Department of Health, Education, and Welfare. *Vocational Rehabilitation: Program Analysis 1967–13.* Washington, D.C., 1967. p. 37.

making decisions that will take effect in the future, there is inevitably a large element of the third factor, uncertainty. This can be dealt with in several ways, the most useful of which is sensitivity analysis. Sensitivity analysis allows the decision maker to change key factors in the analysis to see what the impact of such variation would be.

Time Value of Money: Many health goals can be reached by several means, and frequently these means have significantly different time-frames (for example, research versus expanded application of existing knowledge). As a result, it is necessary to make intertemporal comparisons, usually through the time value of money, which is computed as a flow of funds discounted at an appropriate interest rate. Once again, this sounds simple, but there is indeed a difficult problem, that is, selection of the proper discount rate. To illustrate that this is not trivial, consider the same disease prevention program which has benefits with a present value of $46 million at a discount rate of 10 percent, and $71 million at a discount rate of 4 percent. Also, it must be remembered that the pattern of cash flow in both programs will have a bearing on how important the rate of discount will be. For example, if, in one program, most costs occur in the immediate future and benefits are not realized for many years, while in another program, the costs and benefits tend to run concurrently, then it can be readily seen that the higher the discount rate the less favorable the first program will appear.

There are three popular interest rates: cost of government borrowing, rate of return on private investments (not a unique value), and weighted-average, market interest rate that individuals would receive on the money they use to pay taxes.[29] Even among economists, however, there is little agreement in this area, as shown by the fact that various studies use interest rates that vary from 0 to 9 percent. It is generally considered necessary to use a low rate of return when evaluating public projects, since people tend to undervalue the needs of future generations. Such a low interest rate encourages the acceptance of many government proposals and, thus, forces saving for the benefit of future generations. The interesting question is whether or not this is wise, in view of the fact that, because of our continuing pattern of economic growth, future generations will certainly be richer than the present generation. Baumol[30] suggests that the interest rate should be kept high to

[29] Feldstein, Martin S. "Opportunity Cost Calculations in Cost-Benefit Analysis." *Public Finance,* *19*(2):120, 1964.
[30] Baumol, William J. "On the Social Rate of Discount." *American Economic Review,* *58*(4):799, September 1968.

discourage excessive government investment projects, and that the money thus saved should be diverted to consumption projects to help those who are currently in need. Professor Machlup[31] also urges higher rates for government projects. His contention is that, given the trend toward greater government involvement in everyday life, the use of a low discount rate could eventually lead to the government undertaking a great variety of commercially unprofitable projects while the private sector was deprived of funds. This is, of course, a restatement of the opportunity cost argument.

The government is now struggling with the problem of setting a standard interest rate for use by all federal agencies. It is hard to be sanguine about the outcome of this endeavor because of the political factors involved. To illustrate this point, it has been noted that every water project would be dropped if even the low rate of government borrowing were used as a criterion; this action, of course, would never be tolerated by either the legislative or executive branches because of political implications.[32] Similarly, the proponents of highway construction have succeeded in getting legislation passed which requires the Department of Transportation to use very low interest rates.[33]

Even when discount rates have been established, this is not the end of the problem, because they must still be adjusted to compensate for changes that can reasonably be expected to occur during the life of the project. For example, in a study on chronic kidney disease, the discount rate was adjusted to show a change in productivity because of technological changes in dialysis. Interestingly enough, a different discount rate was used for hospital dialysis than that used for home dialysis.[34] This implies that home dialysis methods will change less than hospital techniques or that the labor of family members in performing home dialysis is free. Klarman,[35] whose method has been followed quite consistently in HEW studies, also makes an adjustment

31 Machlup, Fritz. "Comments on 'Preventing High School Dropouts.'" In: Dorfman, Robert, ed. *Measuring Benefits of Government Investments.* Washington, D.C., The Brookings Institution, 1965. p. 156.
32 U.S. Congress, Joint Economic Committee, Subcommittee on Economy in Government, 90th Congress, 1st session. Hearings on September 14, 19, 20, and 21, 1967. *The Planning-Programming-Budgeting-System: Progress and Potentials.* Washington, D.C., U.S. Government Printing Office, 1967. p. 160.
33 Banks, Robert L. and Kotz, Arnold. "The Program Budget and the Interest Rate for Public Investment." *Public Administration Review,* 26(6):283–292, December 1966.
34 U.S. Bureau of the Budget. "Report of The Committee on Chronic Kidney Disease." September 14, 1967. (Unpublished Report)
35 Klarman, Herbert E. "Syphilis Control Programs." In: Dorfman, Robert, ed. *Measuring Benefits of Government Investments.* Washington, D.C., The Brookings Institution, 1965. p. 403.

for increases in medical costs. His study of syphilis is one that showed a 0-percent rate of interest. It appears that he started with a positive discount rate and arrived at 0 percent as a result of adjustments for cost increases.

Price Changes: Any historical monetary data used to estimate costs or benefits must be adjusted to a common value, preferably current dollars. The common practice is to make such an adjustment using the consumer price index (CPI), but this type of adjustment is totally inappropriate for the health care delivery system. For example, in recent years, physicians' fees have risen faster than the CPI by 1.25 percent per year, and the cost of hospitalization has risen 4 percent per year faster. Because of uncorrected deficiencies in its original construction and problems of differences in the quality of care, the medical care price index is even more vulnerable to criticism than is the price index for almost any other class of commodity. Scitovsky[36] argues that much of the difficulty arising from changes in methods of medical care could be eliminated by a shift from pricing inputs (for example, drugs, X-rays, etc.) to pricing outputs (for example, appendectomy, cure of a streptococcal infection, etc.). This is true, but as Barzel[37] points out, it still does not solve the quality problem. In other words, no really satisfactory technique remains for making the necessary price adjustments; therefore, each analyst will have to choose the one method that most appeals to him. It is important for the decision maker to understand this, so that he can insist upon consistency in analyses of competing projects.

Uncertainty: There are several ways for the decision maker to consider the impact of these choices, of the assumptions made in establishing the ground rules for the study, and of the uncertainties about the parameter estimates used in determining models of alternatives. The primary concern of the analyst is to make it abundantly clear in the report that uncertainties do exist and what the effects of these uncertainties might be. There are at least four ways to do this. The first—probably the easiest and also the least satisfactory—is to include a qualitative discussion of the uncertainties. The second allows the analyst to make a likelihood estimate, that is, to indicate the probability that certain conditions will prevail. Again, this tends to be a rather subjective approach. The third permits a range of possibilities to be

[36] Scitovsky, A.A. "Changes in the Costs of Treatment of Selected Illnesses, 1951–65." *American Economic Review,* *57*(5):1182–1195, December 1967.
[37] Barzel, Yoram. "Costs of Medical Treatment: Comment." *and* Scitovsky, A.A. "Costs of Medical Treatment: Reply." *American Economic Review,* *58*(4):936–940, September 1968.

presented. For example, a kidney disease program analysis[38] used high and low cost assumptions for each treatment modality. The high data were based on an assumption of no change from today's methods, and the low data assumed technological advances. At the end of the fifth year, the range was from $1 billion to $1.5 billion; after 15 years, the range was from $1.8 billion to $2.8 billion. Similarly, in analyzing programs for delivering health services to the poor, HEW felt it was necessary to use high and low estimates because they had no assurance that the target population would utilize fully the services made available to it.[39] Often these estimates provide three levels: optimistic, most probable, and pessimistic.

The fourth and last approach is really a variant of the third. It is called sensitivity analysis[40] and is designed to show how much the outcome is affected by a change in some factor. If, for example, a 20-percent change in a parameter caused only a 1-percent change in the end result, the analyst and the decision maker could conclude that the system was relatively insensitive to that parameter; thus, even a large degree of uncertainty in estimating its value would not be especially dangerous. This approach is surely better than the others in terms of what it can do with regard to displaying the degree of uncertainty; moreover, the degree of sensitivity will indicate the level of accuracy and precision that should be sought in gathering data concerning the parameter.

This concludes the discussion on the several methods of evaluating alternatives by using cost-benefit techniques. The final section of this chapter will cover the implications of such evaluations when the health care administrator is making decisions on the basis of cost analyses.

IMPLICATIONS FOR HEALTH CARE ADMINISTRATORS

It is obvious to all that planning, either compulsory or voluntary, is fast becoming a fact of life in the health care field. A major function in the

38 Kidney Disease Program Analysis Group. "Kidney Disease Program Analysis: A Report to the Surgeon General." Washington, D.C., U.S. Public Health Service, 1967. p. 31. (Unpublished Report)
39 U.S. Department of Health, Education, and Welfare. *Delivery of Health Services for the Poor: Program Analysis 1967–12.* Washington, D.C., 1967. p. 56.
40 Technically, sensitivity analysis studies only the effect of changes in key parameters. Changes in assumptions are assessed by contingency analysis, but the concept is the same for both.

planning process is formulating alternative ways to achieve desired objectives and then choosing between these alternatives. In the past, these choices have been made on the basis of unguided intuition and judgment. Cost-benefit analysis will not replace intuition and judgment, but it can aid the decision maker in a number of ways. These include more precise definitions of objectives, identification of criteria for judging results, quantification of the results of each alternative, formal exposition of assumptions, and examination of the effects of assumptions and uncertainties. In other words, cost-benefit analysis provides a more solid basis for the exercise of judgment.

This technique has been successfully applied in the health care field, and there is ample evidence that it will become an accepted, even mandatory, method of decision making throughout the public sector. Thus, regardless of his personal views about quantitative methods, the health care administrator can confidently expect that he will have to employ this technique in order to obtain support for any significant publicly financed project he wishes to undertake; furthermore, as he progresses to higher levels of administration, he will be called upon to make decisions on the basis of cost-benefit analyses. The foregoing discussion presented a general overview of this method and covered several points in some detail. The administrator should use this material as a point of departure from which to develop the necessary expertise in the use of this technique. He should also become familiar with the problems that have impeded its use in the health care field and begin working toward solutions, so that the full power of this method can be obtained in the future.

These impediments fall into three categories: data, standards, and training; they are neither mutually exclusive nor sequential. Efforts to solve them can go on concurrently and, because of the long-term nature of these problems, must begin at once.

DATA

The data problem, discussed in a later section of this chapter, appeared in virtually all phases of the development of cost-benefit analysis. It is generally agreed that there are many gaps in the available information about the health care system as it exists in the United States today. It is significant to note, however, that the requirements of cost-benefit analysis highlight these deficiencies. The quality of any analysis is directly dependent upon the quality of the data used.

The long lead-time problem is especially critical because, even after a suitable data system is established, it will take years to accumulate the information required for longitudinal studies. Obviously, the first step is to inform those who are designing data systems of exactly what data are required, and this can be done best on the basis of actual experience. One way to accomplish this task is to have managers begin making cost-benefit analyses at once, so that information requirements can be more precisely identified. Requirements thus identified can be defined in terms of classes of data; also, formats can be developed for recording the data (for example, cost data will be needed, and they must not be accumulated in the traditional accounting style). Another technique to improve the usability of data is to avoid aggregation. When details are available, it is possible to develop any kind of summary; but it is impossible to disaggregate a summary so that the details can be restructured into another statistic. The feasibility of this approach will continue to improve as the cost of computerized storage decreases and data processing speed increases.

STANDARDIZATION

One of the great deficiencies in today's data system design efforts is failure to provide for interface between systems. For example, plans for a partial health data system have been made for at least one city without apparent regard for what is being done in other parts of the SMSA. Standardization of data elements (definitions) and codes is a minimum requirement for the transfer of information from one system to another. The health administrator must insist upon this, for all systems reporting to his system and for all related systems (for example, welfare) that operate at the same level. Also, it will be to his advantage to try to make his system compatible with any external system to which he must furnish information. This is important for two reasons: First, it will facilitate the reporting of data. Second, it will allow him to draw data from the other systems for use in his own analyses.

Since cost-benefit analyses often involve a choice among competing proposals, the decision maker should establish standardized adjustment procedures at the outset, so that all data presented to him will be consistent. When he is in the position of making intermediate decisions (for example, acting as a state official selecting local proposals to compete at the national level for grant money), he must be prepared to fight for the adjustment factor he has selected in the event the ultimate decision maker fails to set standards. For example, if California consistently used a 4-percent discount rate and New York used 9 percent, the projects selected by one state would probably have a different cash flow pattern than those selected by the other state. Depending upon the rate used in the federal evaluation process, one or the other would have a great advantage in the competition.

Actually, if procedures are thoroughly standardized, and analyses are performed by mathematical models programmed for computers, the health administrator, acting as the ultimate decision maker, would have the option of replicating all competing analyses using factors of his own choosing. It may be difficult to obtain this degree of standardization at the national level, but insofar as the states are concerned, it is easier to conceive of an aggressive state health agency using its authority and control of funds as levers to establish and enforce statewide standards.

TRAINING

Not every health administrator will become a cost-benefit analyst, but all those who will be involved in any significant use of public funds must understand the cost-benefit technique at least as well as accounting systems are now understood. Cost-benefit analysis is not a gimmick. Formal economic analysis is becoming a way of life for the health care field. Thus, administrators must have a firm grasp of its fundamental concepts, and at least a conversational familiarity with its techniques. This need can perhaps be met by diligent self-study and/or short workshop training sessions.

Health planners, however, must have a much more comprehensive knowledge of the subject. In particular, they must be familiar with systems techniques, especially the construction of models. Without these models, much of the power of the cost-benefit technique will be lost. The easiest way to achieve this level of expertise would be through formal academic course work. Unfortunately, the demand for analysts is already far greater than could be produced over a period of several years. The most likely solution to meet this shortage appears to be by employing those methods used in the data processing field: hire a few technical experts (econometricians) and put them to work with highly talented, functional specialists (health administrators) who have a good fundamental knowledge of economic concepts. In the process of working together, each group will acquire some of the skills of the other, and, eventually, each individual who is exposed to this dual training method will become capable of operating as an independent, health-oriented, cost-benefit analyst.

THE DATA PROBLEM

In discussing model building, cost measurement, and benefit measurement, it was pointed out that the lack of necessary data is a serious limitation to the accomplishment of cost-benefit analyses. Model building and other types of analysis will be easier, and the outputs will be more reliable, if the quality and quantity of health data are improved. It should be noted that the ability to relate health data to other socioeconomic and demographic data will be important. Unless this capability is built into the data system, there will be incomplete analyses or redundant files. Other problems that must be met are standardization of definitions and formats and determination of how to deal with changes that occur over time. It is fairly easy to visualize standard data elements and codes and the adjustment of monetary data by the use of price indexes; but in a longitudinal study, how should we disaggregate early data that grouped into one category several illnesses which are now considered to be distinct entities?

The lack of data on diseases that plagued the earliest studies has not improved much even today. For example, lack of information on heart disease and alcoholism forced HEW to abandon its plans to conduct analyses in these areas even though data on heart disease obviously would have been of interest to President Johnson.[41] The programs of the National Center for Health Statistics are a major effort to help overcome the lack of data on diseases, but they have too many shortcomings. NCHS's data, for example, can be used to obtain estimates of losses due to death and illness, but not losses due to debility resulting from illness. Most important, it does not produce the small-area data required for areawide health planning.

Cost data are even more difficult to obtain than are disease statistics. Data on hospital costs are available from a number of sources, but they are not especially useful. At the individual hospital level, there are very little suitable cost data, because most administrators lack the sophistication to recognize the need for anything beyond accounting data. As noted previously, the Hospital Administrative System (HAS) also collects accounting data; however, this is of dubious value because the recommended allocation bases can provide varying allocations even when total cost is the same, and there is no way of determining comparability of outputs. Although Lave's[42] excellent

41 Drew, Elizabeth B. "HEW Grapples with PPBS." *Public Interest,* 7:11, Summer, 1967.
42 Lave, Judith R. "A Review of the Methods Used to Study Hospital Costs." *Inquiry,* 3(2):57–81, May 1966.

review of hospital cost studies reports that the methods used vary from verbal descriptions, through manipulation of accounting data, to complex statistical techniques, it is difficult to find many of the latter. NCHS has plans to add patient charge information to its data base, but this also will be couched in the usual accounting forms and, of necessity, will be limited to hospitalized patients. It is hard to imagine a system that would adequately cover outpatient costs in the present health system. Medicare data on the over-65 population might help. Another special population group on which some data will become available are the medically indigent who are treated under Medicaid; however, these will be reported by the more than 50 separate systems for administration of the one program. The same problem of diversity, of course, prevails with health insurance data.

Almost every state's proposal for its comprehensive health planning program includes establishment of a data base as a major objective, but whether this will materialize is uncertain. Some interviews indicate that health planners are procrastinating in the hope that some other agency will build a data base which they can use. Further, even those states that have begun to deal with this problem have seldom gotten beyond the point of devising recurring reports based upon data in existing files.[43] An interesting issue here is the level at which the data should be collected and aggregated for most efficient use. For example, New York City reports that it has begun collecting its own health data because national and even state aggregations mask unique characteristics of the local area.[44] In short, it is apparent that the nature and extent of the problem have been generally recognized, and that several of the more progressive states or communities have initiated programs to deal with it. These programs are often based upon concepts of statistical reporting that limit their usefulness, in contrast to the utility of a general purpose data base comprised of disaggregated records. Moreover, there is little likelihood that the data from these various individual programs will be sufficiently compatible to permit aggregation and summarization of data from several systems, as would be required in planning for an SMSA that crosses state boundaries. The Federal Government, however, also has recognized the problem and has developed a positive program for dealing with it. This effort to develop a federal-state-local health statistics system seeks to ensure the availability of data that will be sufficiently detailed for use at the community level and

[43] Derry, John R. et al. "California Health Information for Planning Service." *Inquiry*, 5(3):58–63, September 1968.
[44] Densen, Paul M. et al. "Research, Program Planning, and Evaluation." *Public Health Reports*, 81(1):49–56, January 1966.

sufficiently standardized to allow aggregation of the data that are required at state and national levels. This system, however, is being developed on a cooperative basis which suggests that change will be gradual. Thus, it seems reasonable to predict that it will be a rather long time before a fairly complete nationwide health data system becomes a reality.

The analyst, however, should not give up in despair. Some of the most sophisticated analytic organizations in the country frequently use a data base consisting of files of technical papers, statistical reports, congressional hearings, periodicals, articles, etc. As the George Washington University's State-Local Finance Project has discovered, a great deal can be done by improvising with data that are available in existing public and private files.[45] They may not be the ideal data, but they can produce approximate answers that are far superior to the product of unguided intuition. To illustrate this point, even faced with the limitations we have mentioned, there have been many recent reports of useful models developed in such diverse areas as: effects of a malaria control program on a national economy;[46] regional coordination of use of OB facilities;[47] effectiveness of periodic examinations;[48] returns to scale of group practice;[49] demand for health services;[50] need for bed allocation;[51] locational efficiency of hospitals;[52] and effectiveness of preventive health programs.[53]

CONCLUSION

Cost-benefit analysis has been demonstrated as a useful technique in the health care field. There are many obstacles to the use of some of its more

45 The George Washington University, State-Local Finance Project. *PPB Notes 1 through 11.* Washington, D.C., undated. p. 5.

46 Barlow, Robin. "The Economic Effects of Malaria Eradication." *American Economic Review,* 57(2):130–148, May 1967.

47 Long, Millard F. and Feldstein, Paul J. "Economics of Hospital Systems: Peak Loads and Regional Coordination." *American Economic Review,* 57(2):119–129, May 1967.

48 Lincoln, Thomas L. and Weiss, George H. "A Statistical Evaluation of Recurrent Medical Examinations." *Operations Research,* 12(2):187–205, March–April 1964.

49 Yett, Donald E. "An Evaluation of Alternative Methods of Estimating Physicians' Expenses Relative to Output." *Inquiry,* 4(1):3–27, March 1967.

50 Wireck, Grover C., Jr. "A Multiple Equation Model of Demand for Health Care." *Health Services Research,* 1(4):301–346, Winter 1966.

51 Goldman, Jay; Knappenberger, H.A.; and Eller, J.D. "Evaluating Bed Allocation Policy with Computer Simulation." *Health Services Research,* 3(2):119–129, Summer 1968.

52 Schneider, Jerry B. "Measuring the Locational Efficiency of the Urban Hospital." *Health Services Research,* 2(2):154–169, Summer 1967.

53 McCall, J.J. *Preventive Medicine Policies.* Santa Monica, Calif., The RAND Corporation, 1966. p. 3368.

elaborate methods, but a great deal can be accomplished with just the more rudimentary techniques. Moreover, it appears that wider use of cost-benefit analysis will contribute to the solution of these problems.

Cost-benefit analysis is a useful but imperfect tool; however, it should be used even though it lacks perfection. Improvements will occur by an evolutionary process while the users are benefitting from assistance in the solution of their current problems.

CHAPTER 11

EVALUATION

This chapter will offer, first, an explanatory definition of evaluation and, then, will relate the principles inherent in the definition to the health field.

Evaluation may be defined as a process that determines the results attained by some activity which was designed to accomplish a valued goal or objective. Evaluation fits the model of research because it involves determination of the relationships between a stimulus, which is the program, and the outcome, which is the result, in terms of measurable criteria derived from values. In concept, evaluation tests a hypothesis which supposes that the program causes the desired result. Ideally, in performing evaluation, the typical research design should be followed. In an operational setting, however, sometimes it is not practical to do this exactly; nevertheless, the evaluative design should come as close as possible to a research design.

PURPOSES OF EVALUATION

In general, there are two reasons for having an evaluation program. First, the resources for conducting any activity are limited, and we want to be assured that these limited resources are being used in the best possible fashion and, at the same time, are achieving the desired ends. Second—and this is especially important in the health field—the effects of decisions often are irreversible; therefore, we must know as quickly as possible whether or not the outcomes are what we anticipated. For example, we are unable to resurrect a person who dies because of a misconceived health services program.

More specifically, the major purposes of evaluation[1] can be enumerated as follows:

[1] Suchman, Edward A. *Evaluative Research*. New York, Russell Sage Foundation, 1967. p. 141.

1. Evaluation allows us to measure the effectiveness of a program, that is, the degree to which our objectives are being met.

2. Evaluation allows us to examine the efficiency of the program. Are we getting enough results to justify the amount of resources used?

3. Evaluation, properly used and designed, is a quality control device. It allows us to ensure not only that we are getting quantity, but that the material or services being furnished meet the minimum standards of acceptability.

4. Evaluation enables us to identify side effects. These may be positive or negative, but negative side effects are particularly important in health programs because of the potential hazards involved. Positive side effects will increase the justification for continuing the program.

5. Evaluation helps to identify the strengths and weaknesses in the processes used to carry out the program, so that we can either correct the weaknesses or build upon the strengths.

6. Evaluation not only allows us to test the effectiveness of the program itself, it also permits us to test the effectiveness of the organizational structure and/or the modes of operation. In other words, it is conceivable that a program may be performing unsatisfactorily through no fault of the program per se, but because of organizational deficiencies.

7. Evaluation develops a critical attitude among the program staff, provided the program is properly conceived (for example, so that evaluation is based upon productivity rather than activity). Such an attitude should have positive effects upon performance of the program itself and should stimulate further innovations.

8. Evaluation is a means of providing explicit accountability to the public. This use of evaluation requires an unusual degree of coverage on the part of the program administrator, but, if used with integrity, it can be a valid response to the mounting demands for community awareness and involvement in service programs.

STEPS IN EVALUATION

There are four significant steps in an evaluation process. The first of these—setting of goals—has already been discussed at considerable length in earlier chapters; however, as we proceed through the evaluation process, the necessity for operationalized definitions of goals and selection of explicit criteria will become more and more evident.

The second step is to instrument the process or the program of evaluation; that is, setting up procedures for collecting evaluation data at appropriate points of intervention, storing those data, and then retrieving them when needed.

The third step is to analyze the data which are collected. This analysis should include verbal descriptions of the qualitative factors; quantitative descriptions, such as enumeration statistics, frequencies, and distribution; and, finally, quantitative analyses.

The fourth step is to make the necessary adjustments to the program on the basis of the information obtained from the analyses in step three.

HIERARCHY OF EVALUATIONS[2]

Evaluation of a program is not a single process, but, rather, a number of evaluations which can be arranged in a hierarchy. This hierarchy consists of three levels; the recipient of the service, the provider of the service, and the researcher for the program. For each of these levels, there are three types of evaluation: immediate, intermediate, and long range; and for each type, there are five categories of evaluation. Figure 14 illustrates this hierarchy of evaluation.

LEVELS OF EVALUATION

The level of evaluation will determine the values that are applied; thus, level becomes a key issue. For example, the recipients of a service may tend to emphasize intuitive reactions to outcomes. The provider of a service will express professional concern with efficiency and standards. The researcher for a program is typically a distant, disinterested third party who will employ a scientific methodology in its purer forms for the purpose of gaining knowledge rather than for managing or controlling a program.

TYPES OF EVALUATION

The type of evaluation—immediate, intermediate, or long-range—determines which variables can be measured by evaluation.

2 Many of these concepts were developed and presented by Suchman (see footnote 1). They have been revised and substantially restructured in the presentation. The reader who wishes to compare this suggested framework with the earlier version, should consult Suchman, pp. 51–73.

LEVEL	I. RECIPIENT OF SERVICE	II. PROVIDER OF SERVICE	III. RESEARCHER
TYPE	A. Immediate	A. Immediate	A. Immediate

CATEGORY	1. Effort
	2. Effect
	3. Impact
	4. Efficiency
	5. Process
	   a. Attributes
	   b. Recipients
	   c. Conditions
	   d. Effects
	     (1) Number
	     (2) Duration
	     (3) Type
		Same categories as Recipient of Service	Same categories as Recipient of Service

TYPE	B. Intermediate	B. Intermediate	B. Intermediate
CATEGORY	Same categories as Immediate	Same categories as Immediate	Same categories as Immediate
TYPE	C. Long-Range	C. Long-Range	C. Long-Range
CATEGORY	Same categories as Immediate and Intermediate	Same categories as Immediate and Intermediate	Same categories as Immediate and Intermediate

Figure 14:   Levels, types, and categories of evaluation

The immediate type of evaluation typically covers a period of zero to three years. An example of the type of outcome that can be measured at this level would be improvement of knowledge, which should reduce disinterest, or of acceptability, which should reduce dissatisfaction.

The intermediate level of evaluation typically covers a period of three to five years. Examples of what might be measurable within this time span are signs of improved health, a reduced morbidity rate, or a reduced discomfort threshold.

Long-range evaluation occurs at any time after the end of the intermediate period. At this level, we are interested in measuring those phenomena that become apparent only after the passage of a considerable length of time. For example, in the health field, we would not expect to see much difference in life expectancy until a good many years have passed.

It should be noted, however, that all of the evaluations described above deal with output. To reiterate what was discussed in Chapter 5 on goals and objectives, our concern is with productivity and not with activity. In other words, we are interested in results and not in intermediate inputs. Nevertheless, it is possible to do some sort of evaluation before output (effects) becomes apparent. This is possible because we have theoretical bases which give us an ability to predict probable outcomes given certain conditions. Although this kind of evaluation tends to be administrative in nature, it can be quite effective. First, program inputs can be analyzed with the realization that they are a necessary, albeit not a sufficient, condition to achieve output. Thus, we are concerned with service statistics on where, when, and how many. Second, the program design can be assessed to see if there are any organizational or administrative flaws that may be fatal. For example, we are concerned with the organizational structure, staffing of the organization, plans for sustained funding, relationships with other agencies, and whether or not the organization has already established internal evaluation procedures. The last question, in essence, is asking whether or not the organization has made arrangements for immediate feedback that will allow it to make appropriate adjustments to the program as soon as deviations are detectable.

CATEGORIES OF EVALUATION

The next rank in the hierarchy of evaluations has been designated as categories. There are five of these.

The first category is *effort*. This, to some extent, overlaps what was discussed in the preceding section of this chapter as the analysis of inputs, because here we are dealing with the quantity and the quality of activity. There is an assumption, of course, that activity leads to productivity.

The second category is *effect*. This is a measurement of the result of activity, which confirms or refutes the assumptions made in the earlier category.

The third category is *impact* or *adequacy*. This measures the degree to which effective performance is adequate for total needs. A program could be very effective if it concentrated all its resources on a small segment of the population. Nevertheless, such a program would be judged as totally inadequate. Often, impact is expressed as the product of effectiveness and the number of people exposed. To explain this point, if a 50-percent effective program serves 1,000 people, the result is that 500 people benefit; if a 10-percent effective program is applied to 10,000 people, then 1,000 people will benefit. Consequently, the latter would be preferred, since a greater number of people would be positively affected by the activity.

The fourth category is *efficiency*. This is analogous to a cost-benefit analysis; that is, it is a ratio of the effect (benefit) to the effort (cost). It is usually expressed in terms of cost per unit, with an implied question about the reasonableness of that cost.

The fifth category is *process*. Basically, this is an analysis of how and why the program works. The process evaluation will tend to show the reasons for success or failure. There are four subdimensions of this particular category.

1. The attributes of the program, its organization, its staffing, and its funding.

2. A description of the recipients of the program: Who does this program reach? Who does it not reach? What kind of people are they? One could hardly expect to achieve a high degree of effectiveness, for instance, with a birth control program among a population that has religious scruples against such procedures.

3. The condition under which the program operates: the locale, the timing, and the auspices are the critical issues here. To illustrate this point, a rural health program has substantially different problems than one which is operated in an urban setting. Also, a program that functions under the auspices of a medical society can expect different acceptance than one which is organized by a consumer group.

4. The effects of the program. In this case we are concerned with the character of the objectives that the program seeks to obtain. For example: Are we seeking a unitary goal, or do we seek multiple benefits? How long do we expect these effects to endure? A health education program seeking to persuade people to obtain immunizations in the face of an incipient epidemic is confronted with different problems than a program encouraging people to give up smoking for a lifetime. Finally, the type of effects sought is important. Are we seeking cognitive effects, that is, to change people's thought patterns? Are we seeking attitudinal effects, that is, to change their values? Are we seeking behavioral effects, that is, to change their actions?

The categories of evaluation are very well explained and illustrated by Dr. George James' analogy of a bird.[3] The first category, *effort*, asks: "How

[3] James, George. "Planning and Evaluation of Health Programs." In: Confrey, Eugene A., ed. *Administration of Community Health Services*. Chicago, International City Managers' Association, 1961. p. 126.

many times did it flap its wings?" The second category, *effect*, asks, "How far did the bird fly?" The next, *adequacy* or *impact*, asks, "How far did the bird fly in relation to the length of its total journey?" The fourth category, *efficiency*, asks, "Was there a shorter route?" And, finally, *process* asks, "How does the anatomy of the bird enable it to fly?"

INSTRUMENTATION

Now that we have seen the hierarchy of evaluation, we must turn our attention to the problem of instrumentation, that is, the process of obtaining the data which are necessary to meet the requirements of that hierarchy.

Under ideal circumstances, the data required for evaluation, particularly the quantitative data, should be obtained from the operating system of the program. Unless this can be done, many risks of inconsistency and incompatibility between the two sets of data will ensue; also, there will probably be some irreconcilable differences between the evaluator and the administrator of the program, with each one insisting that the results he obtained are the correct ones. Frequently, the operating program will not capture the denominator data which are necessary in order to establish rates and to measure impact; however, if the operating program is properly designed, its data will be compatible with information collected by systems designed and operated for other programs. These programs need not be part of health agencies; often the health agency can rely upon some other governmental agency, such as a planning commission, for population data. Obviously, it is much less expensive to make one's own program data compatible with the denominator data than it is to capture and maintain both sets of data as part of the operating program.

If possible, qualitative data from consumers should also be captured as part of the operating program. It is important to avoid the loss or distortion of information that generally takes place when recall is relied upon. People simply do not remember very well, and the greater the period of time that elapses between the event and the inquiry, the greater the decay in the quality of the information obtained.

Qualitative data from professionals can be obtained in two ways. First, they may make direct observations by site visits. Second, they can obtain data through the analysis of records. This latter procedure is fairly common in the health field, particularly in connection with peer review systems and medical audits.

PROBLEMS IN THE DESIGN OF EVALUATION

There are certain significant problems that must be considered in the design of an evaluation process. Five of these are worthy of particular attention.

The first concerns the standard research design, where one would hope to have a control group; however, if we have a health program that presumably improves the status of people, then how can one select those people who are to be deprived of the anticipated benefits? Also, when dealing with people, and particularly when dealing with communities, it is quite difficult to establish similarity between the control group and the experimental group. To some extent, this problem can be overcome by randomized selection, provided there is a large enough population with which to deal.

The second problem involves holding constant the program operator effects, to be sure that only program effect is being measured. In other words, one must be sure that, if a service is rendered to a group of people, all of the service providers (program operators) are of approximately equal qualifications.

Third, it is important to keep both the observers and the observed unaware of the status of the observed persons, so the results will be unbiased. This problem can generally be resolved by use of the placebo technique or other research designs, such as a double blind experiment. Regardless of what technique or design is used, however, one must also be aware of the potential Hawthorne effect on the observed persons. This is a situation in which the persons observed may react atypically simply because they are aware that they are under scrutiny.

The fourth problem relates to the selection of criteria (again, this was discussed to some extent in Chapter 5, on goals). But, to reiterate certain crucial points, we must remember that measurability is not the same as validity. Getting valid measurements of effect is frequently the most troublesome part of designing an evaluation program, but this issue must not be compromised. Also, there is the matter of determining whose standards will be used. Finally, as mentioned earlier, we must concern ourselves with the measurement of outputs or results, rather than with intermediate inputs.

The fifth major problem in the design of evaluation is to develop a specification for the type of action to be taken when standards are not met. This may appear to be a trivial question. If the standard is not met, then should one take corrective action? The answer to that is probably "no." A little reflection will show how complex this issue can become. For example, assume that a standard is set at 75 percent. Unit A produces at 77 percent and Unit B produces at 73 percent. Which of the two has better performance? If we assume that A's performance is better, what do we do with the low performer? Certainly, we cannot take the resources away from the high performer in order to reinforce the activity of the low performer without, in some manner, jeopardizing the level of productivity and the degree of enthusiasm attained by the high performer.

SYSTEMS EVALUATION[4]

Thus far, we have discussed the goal-attainment model of evaluation; however, this is only one of two possible evaluation modes. The goal-attainment model, as the name implies, concerns itself solely with results achieved by a specific program in terms of what that program was required to do. In this connection, there are three factors that must be considered in evaluating the goal-attainment model. First, the goal-attainment model does not consider the resource requirements for organizational maintenance; that is, some things must be done in order to keep the organization viable. Unless there is a viable organization, one cannot have a program; therefore, a certain amount of resources must be committed to such functions as recruiting and training.

Second, the goal-attainment model is likely to be suboptimal, in that it considers only its own goals and does not look to the achievement of the total goals of the organization. For example, geriatric patients in a mental hospital may be receiving less care than is called for by the plan's objectives. It may well be that 50 percent of the geriatric patients receive no therapy at all. If, however, the number of aged receiving no therapy is reduced, then the number of young patients who are receiving intensive therapy also will be

4 Schulberg, H.C. and Baker, F. "Program Evaluation Models and the Implementation of Research Findings." In: Schulberg et al., eds. *Program Evaluation in the Health Fields.* New York, Behavioral Publications, Inc., 1969. pp. 562–572.

reduced, unless, of course, the resources are increased. Also, a reduction in the number of young patients might affect the willingness of medical residents to come to the hospital, because geriatric work is extremely unpopular.

Third, the goal-attainment model overlooks the possibilities of joint product; that is, it does not consider those cases in which one activity may contribute to several goals.

An adequately designed systems evaluation process will overcome or minimize all of these differences.

The systems model of evaluation, however, is much more difficult to structure, because it requires analysis of the entire organization and its environment. It recognizes that the organization must do at least four things for survival, namely: achieve its goals and subgoals, coordinate the operation of its subunits, acquire and maintain resources, and adapt to the demands of the environment.

The systems model highlights the two incompatible needs of any organization. The first of these is stability, or the need for getting the job done at a maximum level; and the second is survival, which requires change if the organization is not to become an anachronism. The systems model emphasizes feedback and adaptation. Goal-attainment tends to overlook this mode of adjusting the plan to meet the needs of the real world encountered during implementation. Thus, in the last analysis, the goal-attainment model must be judged inadequate unless it exists as a subset of a systems model of evaluation.

REFERENCES

1. Greenberg, B.G. "Evaluation of Social Problems." *Review of the International Statistical Institute, 36*(3):260–278, June 1968.
2. Morehead, M.A. "Evaluating Quality of Medical Care in the Neighborhood Health Center Program of the Office of Economic Opportunity." *Medical Care, 8*(2): 118–131, March–April 1970.
3. Sparer, G. and Johnson, J. "Evaluation of OEO Neighborhood Health Centers." *American Journal of Public Health, 61*(5):931–942, May 1971.
4. U.S. Department of Health, Education, and Welfare, Health Services and Mental Health Administration, National Institute of Mental Health. *Planning for Creative Change in Mental Health Services: Use of Program Evaluation.* Washington, D.C., 1972. Publication No. (HSM) 71–9057.

AUTHOR INDEX

SUBJECT INDEX